The Secrets of
MINDFUL BEAUTY

*Revolutionary Techniques
in Anti-Aging and Self-Care*

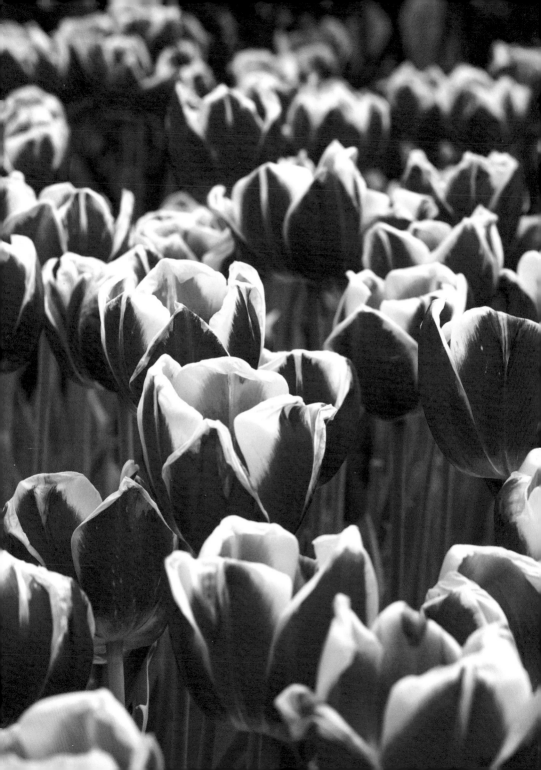

The Secrets of
MINDFUL BEAUTY

Revolutionary Techniques in Anti-Aging and Self-Care

Elizabeth Reid Boyd, PhD
and
Jessica Moncrieff-Boyd, PhD

Photographs by Steve Fraser

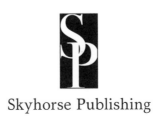

Skyhorse Publishing

Skyhorse Publishing books may be purchased in bulk at special discounts for
sales promotion, corporate gifts, fund-raising, or educational purposes. Special
editions can also be created to specifications. For details, contact the Special
Sales Department, Skyhorse Publishing, 307 West 36th Street, 11th Floor, New
York, NY 10018 or info@skyhorsepublishing.com.

Skyhorse® and Skyhorse Publishing® are registered trademarks of Skyhorse
Publishing, Inc.®, a Delaware corporation.

Visit our website at www.skyhorsepublishing.com.

10 9 8 7 6 5 4 3 2 1

Library of Congress Cataloging-in-Publication Data

Names: Reid Boyd, Elizabeth, 1968- author. | Moncrieff-Boyd, Jessica, author.
Title: The secrets of mindful beauty: revolutionary techniques in anti-aging
    and self-care / Elizabeth Reid Boyd and Jessica Moncrieff-Boyd;
    photographs by Steve Fraser.
Description: New York: Skyhorse Publishing, [2017]
Identifiers: LCCN 2016050244| ISBN 9781510717695 (paperback) | ISBN
    9781510717701 (ebook ISBN)
Subjects: LCSH: Beauty, Personal—Psychological aspects. |
    Aging—Prevention—Popular works. | Stress management—Popular works. |
    Self-esteem in women. | Self-care, Health—Popular works. | BISAC: HEALTH
    & FITNESS / Beauty & Grooming.
Classification: LCC RA776.98 .R45 2017 | DDC 646.7/2—dc23
LC record available at https://lccn.loc.gov/2016050244

Cover design by Jane Sheppard
Cover photo: iStockphoto

Print ISBN: 978-1-5107-1769-5
Ebook ISBN: 978-1-5107-1770-1

Printed in China

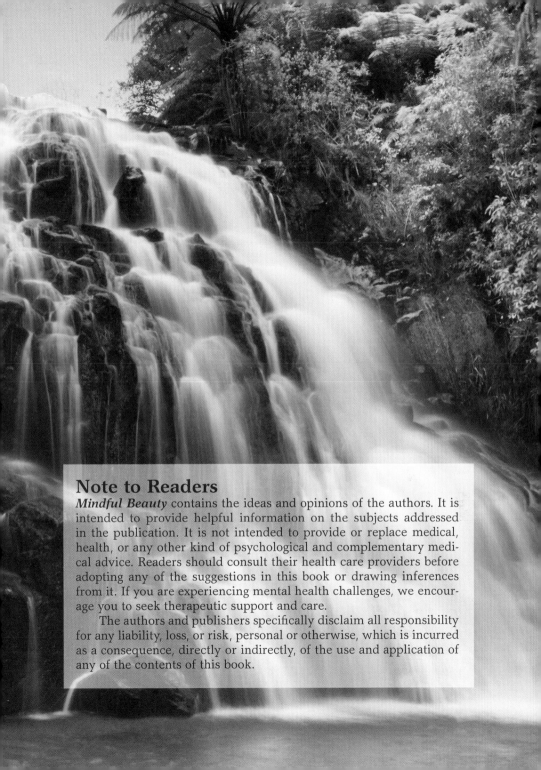

Note to Readers

Mindful Beauty contains the ideas and opinions of the authors. It is intended to provide helpful information on the subjects addressed in the publication. It is not intended to provide or replace medical, health, or any other kind of psychological and complementary medical advice. Readers should consult their health care providers before adopting any of the suggestions in this book or drawing inferences from it. If you are experiencing mental health challenges, we encourage you to seek therapeutic support and care.

The authors and publishers specifically disclaim all responsibility for any liability, loss, or risk, personal or otherwise, which is incurred as a consequence, directly or indirectly, of the use and application of any of the contents of this book.

Contents

Contents

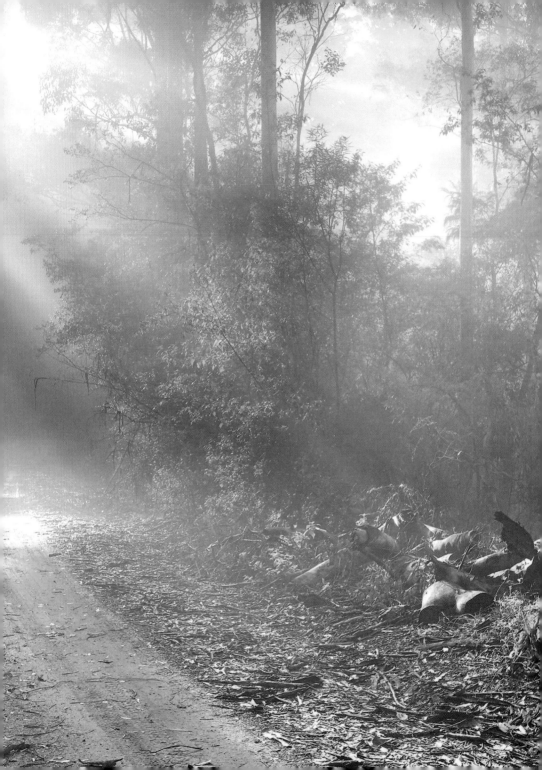

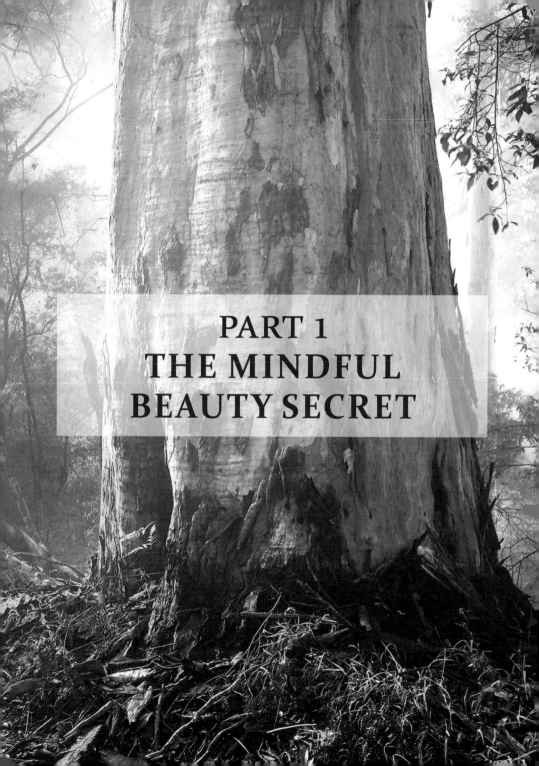

PART 1
THE MINDFUL
BEAUTY SECRET

Introduction: Discover Mindful Beauty

Open your mind to a beautiful new you. Make the mindful beauty connection.

If you think beauty comes from a jar, a salon, or a surgical procedure, think again. The best beauty treatment is in your own mind.

Mindfulness is a hugely popular concept today. You may know that mindfulness can create improvement in our minds and bodies. What you may not know is that mindfulness can also enhance our appearance as well as bring us peace of mind.

Mindful beauty is an exciting method of applying the practices of mindfulness to our overall health and well-being. The unique mindfulness techniques you'll discover in this book offer a brand-new way to bring the benefits of mindfulness into beauty and self-care. Mindfulness can be used to reduce stress and enhance beauty, and in this easy-to-follow guidebook, you'll find out how.

Mindful beauty is about reclaiming the practices of beauty and self-care and turning them into experiences that assist us to be present and accepting of ourselves, our bodies, our thoughts, and our feelings. Too many of our beauty routines are fraught with anxiety, self-criticism, stress, or even self-loathing. There is a way to look and feel better. The revolutionary mindful beauty treatments in this book have been specially created for a happier, more beautiful you.

Changing Our Minds About Beauty

Over the years, there's been a lot of trivialization of women's beauty and self-care. Many women experience embarrassment and shame about the time or money they spend on themselves because they've been told or internalized the idea that it's trivial or superficial. If we're struggling with self-care, poor self-esteem, body distress, feelings of not being good enough, or even if we're just tired or stressed out, the last thing we need to hear is that our worries aren't important or worthwhile. It's time for women to have a more positive, compassionate attitude toward themselves.

That's where mindfulness comes in. Mindfulness can decrease our self-consciousness so that we become less worried about what others think of what we say or do, or how we look. It silences the critical voice inside and facilitates the development of self-compassion. Mindfulness doesn't just ground us; it allows us to see things from a new perspective. By paying attention to ourselves in a new way, mindfulness allows us to perceive more than what is merely on the surface, to still the chatter in our minds, to look around and about, above and beyond, within and without. By going deep, we can rise above being called superficial, or better yet, bring new meaning to it.

Mindful beauty can bring about this change by providing powerful mindfulness methods and supportive self-care routines to balance our lifestyles and improve our overall well-being in a way that won't add more stress to our lives. These easy and effective techniques are uniquely designed to improve our appearance, but they'll also give a sense of empowered calm that we can carry with us wherever we go—and we don't need to make room for it in our cosmetics bag. The treatments are presented in a format that can be easily integrated into any beauty routine.

Let mindful beauty take back the beauty in your life by reminding you of the beauty in each moment and how beautiful you really are.

Why We Need Mindful Beauty

Many of us want to break out of the trap of difficult thoughts and feelings about how we look, but we often don't know how. The problem is, stress and poor self-care can often make matters worse.

Did you know worry can give you wrinkles, insomnia can cause sagging skin, anxiety can increase reddening and skin rashes, and stress can result in acne and hair loss? That's why it's vital we reclaim beauty in a mindful way.

Every day millions of dollars are spent on cosmetic products and procedures, often with disappointing, dissatisfying, and sometimes distressing results. The good news is that the easy, cost-effective mindfulness techniques in this book can make a real difference.

Recent medical and psychological research shows that good mental health is a key to good physical health. How we think and feel affects how we look. Specific mental health challenges have particular impacts on different parts of our bodies, such as our skin and hair. Your total well-being also affects your appearance far more than you realize. If you're not balancing your life, it shows. Poor self-care behaviors can cause cumulative collateral damage.

Reducing stress and anxiety is good for your skin. Our state of mind matters. Luckily, many of the routines around beauty lend themselves to mindfulness and can be practiced in a present, nonjudgmental way. These techniques can enhance your experience and have ongoing positive beautifying effects by reducing stress and anxiety, which affects how you look and feel.

You can lose your permanent frown, smooth your worried brow, and turn your sag lines to smile lines with mindful beauty . . . and change your outlook on life at the same time.

A Mother-Daughter Journey
to Mindful Beauty

Elizabeth's Story

I'm in my forties. As many women of a certain age know, it's a time of change in how we look and can be a challenge. One afternoon, glaring at myself in the mirror, my hands pulling my hair back in a tight ponytail, I gloomily asked my daughter, "Do you think I need cosmetic surgery?"

Jessica rolled her eyes in the way only a daughter can. "You don't need cosmetic surgery. You need cosmetic psychology."

I spun around and seized her by the shoulders. "Cosmetic psychology? What's that? Tell me!"

She laughed. "I don't know. I think I just made it up."

"I need it," I stated.

So began our journey to mindful beauty.

What we found fascinated us.

I'm an author and academic with degrees in psychology and a PhD in gender studies. Jessica has also studied psychology and creative writing, and is following it up with a Masters and PhD in clinical psychology. Together, we've published articles on body image in academic journals, and we have both focused our research on issues that affect women's health and well-being.

For the last five years, we've researched, read, written, and experimented with a range of psychological, sociological, and complementary theories and therapies to do with cosmetic psychology. There's not a lot of research in this newly emerging area, but what there is reveals a strong mind-beauty connection.

We have explored cognitive behavioral therapy, emotion-focused therapy, motivational enhancement therapy, body-mind psychotherapy, and self-acceptance training, as well as other psychological, social, and complementary techniques. We've exchanged books, academic articles, and ideas. Most of all, we've tested it ourselves. We have tried various techniques and compared results to find out what worked and what didn't. Sometimes we perceived a slight change in how we looked and how we felt about how we looked. It was only when we came to mindfulness that we noticed an amazing difference.

When we applied the concept of mindfulness to our beauty regimes, things began to change. I first noticed that instead of feeling stressed and rushed when getting ready for work in the morning, I slowed down and began to enjoy it. Jessica reported the same. As we continued to explore and experiment with mindfulness techniques we became more certain we'd made a discovery. Researching and writing the book became a joy.

I soon shared our discovery with my friends, colleagues, and university students, and many were amazed by the results of simple mindfulness techniques and meditation. "My tension headache has gone," said one student. Another reported a reduction in jaw pain, and others commented on their increased openness and awareness. "For the first time I didn't worry about what other people thought of me," a female student revealed.

Mindfulness made me more self-aware too. I was astonished to realize my lifelong approach to beauty had been anything but beautiful. Before practicing mindful beauty, if I was tired or stressed, my beauty regimes were accompanied by a great deal of self-criticism. I'd berate myself for buying certain cosmetics, or for not buying them. I'd wish I had looked after myself better years before. I'd analyze every flaw.

The Secrets of Mindful Beauty

I'd mentally criticize how I put on makeup. When traveling, I'd scold myself for taking too much in my cosmetics bag, or for forgetting what I needed.

With mindful beauty, this changed. I began to look more kindly at myself. Instead of self-care routines being something I forced myself to do, or critiqued myself for not doing, mindful beauty techniques became a bright spot in my day. Morning and night, I sought out times to practice them. My beauty routines became a special time just for me.

Along the way, I also faced a challenging health crisis. I truly believe that if I had not been practicing mindfulness and been tuning into my body in a powerful new way, it would not have had such a timely, fortunate outcome. For me, mindfulness isn't just life-enhancing, it's lifesaving.

Mindful beauty reminds me, every day, to appreciate the beauty in my life. Now, if I ever get off track, I return to these simple, beautiful processes.

I no longer glare at myself in the mirror.

I smile.

Jessica's Story

Mindfulness caught my attention early on in my clinical training. I was drawn to the basic concepts it embraced, such as adopting a nonjudgmental stance and using meditative strategies in practical ways. When looking into the mindfulness literature, I was able to see the benefits it offered in regard to preventing depression relapse. I could also see how it offered helpful strategies for other common mental health difficulties, such as stress and anxiety.

As a provisional psychologist and PhD student, I was often thrown into highly demanding and stressful situations. It became important for me to find my own way to manage stress. On a wider level, I also wanted to be practicing what I preached. I decided that learning about mindfulness, and engaging in my own mindfulness practice, would be a way to do this.

I began attending focused meditation classes. While living in the United Kingdom as a visiting research fellow, I attended a Buddhist meditation center to learn more about the foundational practices of mindfulness. When delivering mindfulness workshops to adolescent girls, I would excitedly do all the exercises myself, inside and outside classes. Soon I found myself doing these automatically, even creating new mindfulness exercises and sharing them with others. I began to reengage with the natural world and developed a love of gardening. Small chores and routines I used to rush through or become irritated by turned into opportunities to engage, notice, and be interested in a mindful, peaceful way.

When Mom and I began discussing the idea for this book, we realized very quickly how applicable mindfulness was to beauty and skin care routines. We decided to test it ourselves. Suddenly, there were so many more opportunities in the day to be mindful! I noticed things I never had before, like how much I enjoyed the smell of my moisturizer (rose), that washing my hair could be a delightful, sensory experience, and that when I took a closer look at the label, the sunscreen I had been using was six months out of date (I enjoyed selecting a replacement). Over time, mindful beauty became a natural part of my daily practices. I noticed further reductions in my typical stress and anxiety levels, and that I felt (and looked) calmer and more balanced. I also noticed that rather than feeling stressed and rushed at the beginning or end of the day, these moments became refreshingly present-focused and healing. Even basic nighttime cleansing routines became not just about skin care; they became about self-care.

I have always had an interest in promoting the mental health and well-being of girls and women. I've attempted to do this through my research into eating disorders, and see a wonderful opportunity to do this through mindful beauty. So many mental health difficulties among women seem to stem from having a difficult or critical relationship with our bodies and our appearance. Mindful beauty is not about changing our appearance; it is about relating to ourselves in a different, healthier way. Rather than changing the picture, we can change the lens we use to see.

About Mindfulness

Mindfulness is a practice and strategy that initially developed from Buddhist traditions. It has recently received attention in psychological fields and has been found to be a successful way of managing anxiety, stress, and even depression.

To be mindful means to be conscious or aware. When we are practicing mindfulness, we are engaging with the present moment, noticing the feelings, thoughts, and sensations that arise at the time. Often, we can get so caught up in our heads, or in a task, that we lose awareness of ourselves and what is going on around us. Have you ever driven a familiar route, and then realized you can barely remember the experience of reaching your destination? Have you ever grabbed a hurried meal and eaten it in a flash without even really tasting it? This often happens when we are on autopilot, in a state of "doing," or when we are caught up in our own worries and stresses. Mindfulness is a way of re-engaging with our moment-to-moment experiences, a way of switching into "being" and becoming aware of ourselves and our surroundings.

The other focus of mindfulness is to adopt a nonjudgmental stance. This is really about practicing acceptance of any thoughts, feelings, or sensations we experience in the moment. It is normal to apply statements or judgments to experiences; for example, when we feel a breeze, thinking it is "too cold." Mindfulness is about letting go of these judgments and just noticing the cold sensation from the breeze, rather than assessing it. This can be the same with our thoughts and feelings. Rather than noticing we feel stressed or upset and deciding we shouldn't feel that way, a mindful experience would be to acknowledge the presence of these feelings and let them be present in the moment.

Meditation is a crucial part of mindfulness. All meditations help us to focus our attention and awareness, and there are many kinds of meditative techniques. Mindfulness meditations that come from the Buddhist tradition are known as *vipassana,* which means to see things as they really are. It incorporates the concept of impermanence. Nothing stays the same. Change, rather than no change, is what's permanent in life. We can't cling to the past, to the way things used to be . . . or to how we used to look. Following this ancient tradition, mindful beauty encourages us to see ourselves as we really are and disengage from negative self-talk that comes from living in a society focused on youth and body image. With the mindful beauty meditations you'll discover in this book, you'll be encouraged to get in touch with the real you and the beauty within. It will help you accept and embrace the ever-changing you. It will change how you see yourself.

Mindfulness can help us to recognize the warning signs of anxious or depressive thinking so we're able to deal with them better. Imagine visiting with a friend who is a bit down. You wouldn't scold them for being sad or enforce a vigorous cheering up. You'd treat them kindly and accept them as they are, at that moment. You'd give them a hug, hold their hand, or sit quietly by their side. You'd be there for them. Mindfulness teaches us to become that kind of friend to ourselves. Being there for yourself takes practice. Mindful beauty offers a way to learn and practice this self-caring skill, by bringing us back to gentle daily routines that can nurture us right now.

Mindfulness has also been incorporated into psychological treatments for depression as part of mindfulness-based cognitive therapy and assimilated into mental health treatment programs in the United States and the United Kingdom. Mindfulness meditations have been found to prevent the return of depressive episodes. It teaches how to focus on the present, rather than worrying about the future or dwelling unhappily on the past. It helps us not to ruminate, to go over and over (and over) problems in our minds. Rumination can be exhausting. It leads us nowhere, except around and around in ever-decreasing circles. Mindfulness is gentle. It doesn't add a scolding voice, an avoidant mental maneuver, or a denial of how you feel. It helps those who are anxious and distressed accept their experiences as they are. By focusing on our bodies, on our physical sensations, such as breathing, or by mindfully engaging in soothing tasks, it helps us to come back to the present, to slow down and experience our feelings and to accept them, instead of getting stuck in a racing, downward spiral of negative thoughts.

Mindfulness-based cognitive therapy has been scientifically tested and is particularly effective with regard to depressive relapse. This is helpful, because if you have ever struggled with depression at a time in your life, it may return at some stage. By learning some simple mindful strategies and making them part of your daily life, you can engage in beneficial preventative mental health care.

Mindfulness has other benefits. It helps you get into flow with your "stream of consciousness" (a phrase coined by William James, the father of psychology). The stream of consciousness is the flow of your thoughts. Being in flow is linked to creativity. In our experience, and in those of many others, mindfulness increases creativity. Evidence is being gathered in this exciting area of research. Mindfulness helps you to dive deep into your creative well, and to learn to rest while constantly moving in the current of life.

About Mindful Beauty

Mindful Beauty is unique. There is no other book that brings mindfulness into the beauty, self-care, and well-being context.

One of the revered masters of the practice of Buddhist mindfulness is the spiritual leader Thich Nhat Hanh. He suggests that simple acts, like washing the dishes or drinking tea, can be transformed into acts of meditation. *Mindful Beauty* takes this philosophy into the realm of beauty and self-care. It draws on these ancient Buddhist roots of mindfulness and balances it with psychological and scientific advances in the area.

A leader of the contemporary mindfulness psychology movement is Jon Kabat-Zinn, the founder of mindfulness-based stress reduction. He emphasizes the value of coming back to our bodies and our senses over and over again. Kabat-Zinn also recommends finding ways to stabilize our attention and presence amidst our daily activities. For every woman, mindful beauty rituals are the perfect time and place to bring mindfulness to life.

Mindfulness offers us an empowering way to bring meaning to our routines. Ellen Langer, the mother of mindfulness, has carried out decades-long research into mindfulness versus mindlessness. When we are acting automatically, engaged in unthinking habits and routines, we are being mindless, which Langer's research suggests has adverse consequences for aging, as well as our long-term health and well-being. But we can break the cycle. *Mindful Beauty* teaches mindfulness skills in a daily context that you can use for life.

Mindfulness has been applied in other environments. It has been taken up in workplaces in order to increase employee satisfaction and performance and is also gaining attention in the fields of education and learning. With mindful beauty, you will find that you bring your new awareness to other parts of your life too.

Mindfulness is happening now. *Mindful Beauty* is accessible and easy to follow without losing the basis of its philosophy and science. *Mindful Beauty* brings the power of now into every woman's bedroom, bathroom, or beauty routine.

How Mindful Beauty Works

In this book, you'll discover how you can use skin care products and cosmetics in a mindful way that promotes a holistic approach to self-care. Many companies and brands involved in beauty consciously or unconsciously promote mindfulness. Go past the hype and you'll see they can offer ways to awaken your sensory experience.

In the last decade, dermatologists have been increasingly informed by the breakthrough research in this area. The American Psychological Association recently reported that psychodermatology, the study of the mind-brain-skin connection, is gaining strength and support. It's still very new, but there's growing evidence-based research and studies in this area. Dermatologists are now working with psychologists to explore the mind-body connection and the role stress and other psychological conditions can have on our bodies. New treatments are at mind level, not at the surface of our skin.

Mindfulness and psychodermatology are both at the cutting edge of psychological research and treatment. Put them together, and you've got mindful beauty: a breakthrough way of approaching physical and mental health. What's surprising is that it hasn't been tried before.

Mindful beauty provides intervention at a point that matters. Many women struggle with body image problems. Under stress or anxiety, we might find ourselves obsessing over a blemish or a wrinkle. When we feel down, or if we are suffering from low self-esteem or body esteem, we might reduce or even halt our self-care. This creates a cycle that perpetuates poor mental and physical health, and in the long term may become harmful. Mindful beauty is more than skin deep. The mind-body connection is powerful. The smallest act of mindful self-care can have lasting impacts on our well-being.

The Beauty of Ritual

Mindfulness enhances our sense of ritual and order. In Sanskrit, the word "ritual" means visible order. When we give proper attention to our self-care rituals and fully experience them through our senses, it can evoke a spirit of ceremony that's lacking in our contemporary lives.

In days gone by, self-care rituals were given great honor. Bathing, for example, was a highly stylized ritual. In England, there is an ancient "Order of the Bath" that comes from the ceremony of a knight's investiture. On the night before being granted his title, a prospective knight would take a ceremonial bath. This bath had great significance, indicating spiritual and bodily cleansing for a new life ahead. Bathing was also taken seriously by kings and queens. At the Palace of Versailles in France, next to Marie Antoinette's bathroom, is a rest room, a special room where she would rest after the "exhausting" process of taking a bath. Marie Antoinette enjoyed frequent baths and engaged in elaborate self-care and pampering rituals, supported by her perfumer. In Zen Buddhism, cleansing is carried out with care, and part of festive celebrations is a ceremony known as "bathing the Buddha," evoking the idea of physical and spiritual cleansing. We don't need to be as elaborate or exhaustive as the Order of the Bath at the court of Versailles or become Zen Buddhists, but we can reconsider how we cleanse our bodies and souls.

Mindfulness brings back the beauty of ritual to our daily lives. It helps us to focus on the experience of self-care. By being mindful, we can re-create mindless routines into beautiful rituals. We're not saving energy when we rush through the day. Let the rituals of mindful beauty refresh and energize you.

Key Attitudes of Mindful Beauty

There are eight key attitudes at the heart of mindful beauty. They are drawn from the philosophy and psychology of mindfulness and underpin all the practices you will find in this book.

- **Mindful beauty is nonjudgmental.** By approaching our beauty rituals in a new and nonjudgmental way we become less critical about ourselves and how we look.

- **Mindful beauty engages our five senses.** By increasing our appreciation of what we see, smell, touch, hear, and taste, we begin to enjoy our daily self-care routines more and see the benefits.
- **Mindful beauty is kind.** Its methods are soothing and sensitive, a balm to our souls, minds, and bodies. It brings compassion to self-care.
- **Mindful beauty is simple.** It won't ask you to add more to your schedule, but make the most of routines that are already part of your life. It will give you a sense of everyday pleasure and ease.
- **Mindful beauty is meditative.** Its contemplative approach doesn't require you to switch off for an hour, but to go deeper into your daily life, with refreshing results.
- **Mindful beauty is of the moment.** It brings present moment attention to simple rituals, enhancing our experience of the here and now and the miracle of mindfulness.
- **Mindful beauty is healing.** It can heal the scars inflicted by a lack of self-care in the past or stress about the future by bringing peace into the present.
- **Mindful beauty is a skill.** It takes practice to cultivate. Take time to enjoy the process.

How to Use Mindful Beauty

Like the best cosmetics, a little mindfulness goes a long way. There are so many opportunities for mindfulness in your daily beauty routine, and it's easy to make them part of your life. The more you practice these simple, everyday techniques the better you will look and feel. What's more, they're fun!

What Stress Looks Like—You'll first learn to identify the beauty and aging impacts of common psychological stressors and take a simple stress test to see if you're under pressure. See what the cosmetic consequences look like on your face, and be ready to make a mindful change.

Mindful Beauty Treatments—Discover the secrets. These effective, psychological solutions go direct to the cause, based upon mindfulness therapy. The everyday techniques are presented in a simple format that can be easily integrated into your current beauty routine.

Quick Lifts—Fast mindfulness fixes for an instant improvement are also provided throughout the book. These Quick Lifts are easy to learn and can be practiced anytime, anywhere.

Natural Beauty Spots—Throughout the book you'll see uplifting images of nature to give you a mindful beauty boost. Just like stopping to appreciate a sunset, a flower, or a starry night, focusing on these images will help bring you into a more mindful state of being.

Choose the mindful beauty techniques that most appeal to you. You can use the techniques at random or set up a regular schedule. Start slowly. Choose one technique and incorporate it into your beauty regime, then add another, and then a few more. Keep it slow and steady.

You already have a beauty routine; make it a mindful beauty routine and see the beautiful change in you.

Stay mindful. Stay beautiful.

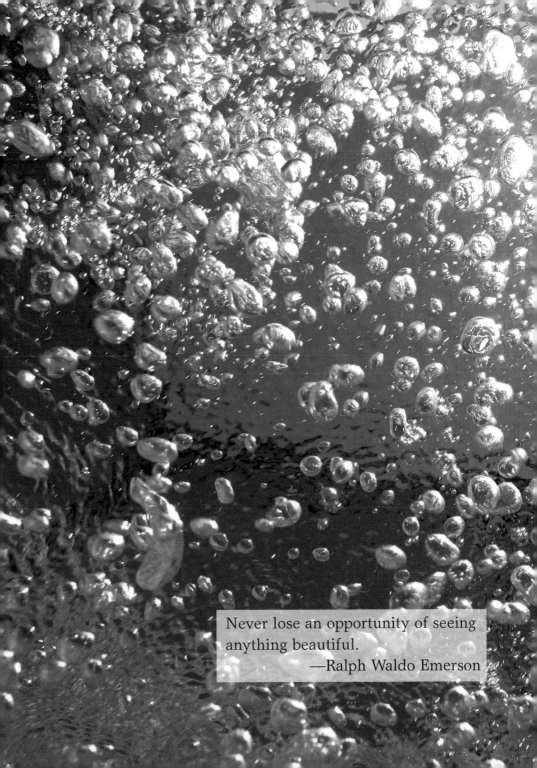

Never lose an opportunity of seeing
anything beautiful.
—Ralph Waldo Emerson

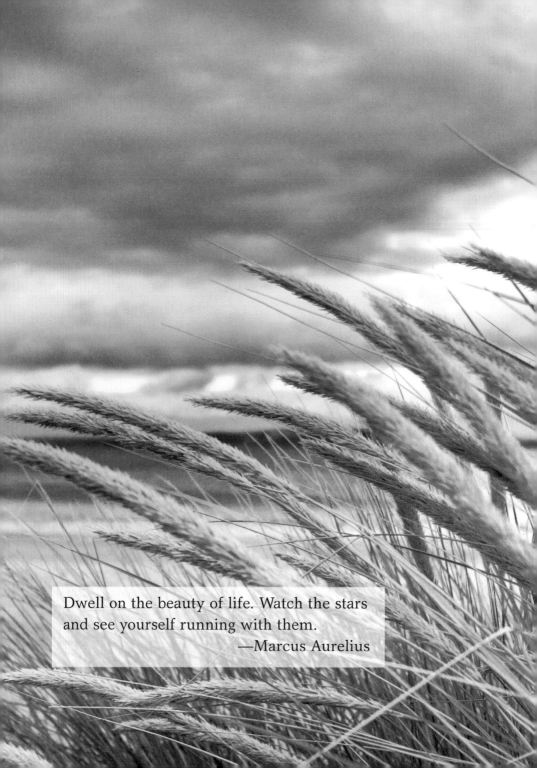

Dwell on the beauty of life. Watch the stars and see yourself running with them.

—Marcus Aurelius

What Stress Looks Like: Take the Test

There are a range of stress factors we all face in life today, no matter what your age. Experiencing stress is a normal response to challenging life events in our work, family, relationships, and other activities. But while stress is part of life, it can get out of hand and has hidden costs on how we look and feel.

There are two kinds of stress. There's positive stress, which gives us energy and makes us productive. Then there's negative stress, which can be debilitating and bad for our minds and bodies.

Positive Stress—With positive stress we enjoy getting up in the morning; we approach our tasks with interest and ease. Our home life runs smoothly, our relationships are good, and we might even love what we're doing so much that we can't believe we get paid to do it! Even if life is busy, we go with the flow and get an energy rush. Positive stress keeps us looking good; we appear vital, excited, and alive.

Negative Stress—When it feels like life is too much for us, we can experience negative stress. We feel overwhelmed, burdened with too much to do, unappreciated, and burned out. We race through the day without stopping, or we give up and just go through the motions. We might also become angry and resentful, and even if we try to keep it inside, we are irritable and easily agitated. We find it hard to relax. This is negative stress, or "di-stress."

Your Body Under Stress

When negative stress kicks in as a response to a challenging event, whether real or imagined, your nervous system releases a flood of stress hormones into your body, including adrenaline and cortisol. Your heart will pound faster, your muscles will tighten, and your blood pressure will rise. You may start breathing more quickly, and your sense of sight, smell, or taste may become sharpened. On the positive stress side, these physical responses are designed to increase your strength and stamina, speed your reactions, and help you to focus and perform better. However, if you are experiencing constant stress overload and negative stress, there will be a heavy cost. You might not notice how much stress you're under anymore; it can creep up on you, and may even feel normal. While a short burst of stress can spur you on to greater things, long-term stress can drag you down, putting a heavy toll on your body and devastating cosmetic effects.

Stress Ages You Faster

A number of scientific investigations have identified more chromosomal changes reflecting cell aging among individuals with higher levels of stress. In one study, women with ongoing life stress had cells that appeared up to ten years older than their chronological age. The physical signs of premature cell aging, such as skin deterioration, can then follow.

Chronic stress can wreak havoc on our appearance. The physical signs of stress, such as frowning, can speed up the development of permanent facial lines and wrinkles. Increased levels of stress hormones, such as cortisol and adrenaline, can lead to acne, hair loss, and poor skin repair. The cosmetic consequences of worry and anxiety are similarly extensive and damaging. Ongoing worry can result in faster wrinkle development, poor skin, and signs of fatigue. Acute attacks of anxiety can result in skin flushing and redness, which has been associated with rosacea.

Facing the Stress Effects
Let's look at the ways stress and anxiety can change our faces.

Stuck in the Groove
Clare was in her mid-twenties when she noticed two vertical lines between her eyebrows that just weren't going away. Though she appears bubbly and outgoing, the truth is, she's a secret worrier. Unfortunately, it has started to show on her face much earlier than she expected. Working in the hair and beauty industry, Clare feels a lot of pressure to look good. She's begun having Botox injections, but is concerned she's going to need the costly treatments for life. She's also concerned about whether they are safe over the long term.

Feelings of worry show on your face. The classic worried look includes a furrowed brow, a pursed or tightened mouth, or a grimace. If a worried facial expression is the norm for you, this might contribute to speeding up line and wrinkle development. According to medical experts, repeated facial expressions result in the formation of grooves under the skin surface. With age, the skin loses elasticity and these grooves can become permanent facial lines and wrinkles.

Locked Jaw
Jenny is in her late fifties. She needs to have expensive dental work done that isn't covered by her health insurance. The reason: at night, she's been grinding her teeth. All the stress she tries to suppress during the day comes out while she's asleep, so in the morning she wakes up with sore teeth and an aching jaw.

Experiencing anxiety can lead to persistent muscle tension, often involving the facial muscles and the jaw. Constant jaw grinding and clenching, known as bruxism, can result in chipped teeth and gum recession that may eventually lead to tooth loss. Jaw clenching and grinding can become an unconscious habit, or it can happen while you sleep.

Tired and Faded

Angelica is starting her career in an accounting firm. As often as she can, she rushes to the bathroom to check her appearance. She frequently touches her face and hair to make sure everything is in place. At lunch time she doesn't like going into the lunch room because she's worried the fluorescent lights makes her look ugly and pale.

Worrying wears you out. Feeling exhausted is a common symptom of anxiety and depression. Ongoing fatigue can arise as an indirect effect of anxiety, sleep problems, and ongoing physical tension and stress. Signs of fatigue show on your face, often in the form of fine lines, dull or dry skin, and dark circles under the eyes.

Red-Faced

Emily has always been easily embarrassed. She was the girl at school who blushed when she had to talk in class. In her thirties, she began to develop a skin condition identified by her dermatologist as rosacea, a reddening of the skin that looks as if she has a permanent rash. This has made Emily even more embarrassed. She's undergoing topical treatments, but she's been told her condition may have an emotional cause.

Facial blushing is a common symptom of anxiety. Flushing and facial redness can also commonly occur during panic attacks. Anxiety-driven blushing and facial redness has been associated with rosacea, a skin condition that involves permanent redness across parts of the face, most commonly the cheeks and forehead. Small blood vessels may also become dilated and apparent under the surface of the skin. In a recent investigation of the causes of rosacea, emotional influences, including stress and anxiety, were listed as the second most prevalent cause of the condition.

Hot and Bothered

Tina's skin is starting to change. She had normal skin for years, but now it has become sensitive and easily inflamed. Food and drink she used to have no problem with are now triggers that leave her unsure of what she can eat, and skin creams that she's used all her life now leave her with a visible rash.

Inflammation is one of the enemies of anti-aging. Skin redness is one of the visible signs of inflammation going on in our bodies, but there's a lot we can't see going on beneath the surface at the cellular level, especially when hormonal change is involved. Medical research reveals that aging inflammation is aggravated by poor diet, but equally problematic is anxiety and stress. Feeling hot and bothered by life can speed the aging process.

Permanent Frown

Laura has a difficult relationship with her mother. One morning she stood under the shower feeling down and anxious about attending a family event, worrying there would be a distressing scene. As she stepped out of the shower, she caught sight of her face in the mirror and realized she was scowling. Her anxiety was written all over her face.

When we're stressed, the tension we feel is revealed in our face. Stress can cause our brow to furrow, our lips to tighten and turn down, and our nose to wrinkle. This might not even be a momentary expression. If you are stressed about being late for an appointment, you might make this kind of face during the whole drive there! According to leading dermatologists, recurrent frowning causes small creases to form under the skin. As we get older, these creases become permanent, leading to lines and wrinkles. Sometimes we can already spot these "hazard" areas. Do you occasionally have small lines along the bridge of your nose? You may regularly wrinkle your nose. Do you sometimes notice two vertical lines between your eyebrows? You may be a brow-furrower. With too much stress, this can become permanent.

Stress Head

When Sasha brushed her hair, she noticed that more and more strands were left in the hairbrush. Her hair looked thin and lank. She visited her GP, who told her hair loss is often caused by stress. Sasha didn't think she'd been under any special stress, but her doctor asked her to cast her mind back to a few months previously, because hair loss often occurs sometime after a stressful situation or event. Sure enough, Sasha had broken up with her boyfriend four months prior.

While strands of our hair are lost every day, sometimes it can fall out thicker and faster than usual. Stress has been identified as one of the leading causes of atypical hair loss. Sometimes as a result of a stressful life event or time period, hair growth becomes dormant and can result in more profuse hair loss two to three months later. This means that if you're experiencing hair loss now, you need to think back a few months to identify the stressful event or trigger that caused it. A more severe form of stress-related hair loss can result in hair falling out in large clumps over the span of a few weeks.

Weak Nails

When Loretta was getting a manicure, her manicurist noticed that Loretta's nails were growing back much weaker than they had previously. Loretta is using false nails to cover the damage, but she's perturbed by what's going on beneath the surface.

Your hands and nails are one of the first places to show the physical effects of stress. Weak, brittle nails have been noted as a common side effect. Habits associated with stress or tension release, such as nail biting and nail picking, can also occur. These habits can often result in rough, ragged nails, broken skin on the nail beds and cuticles, cuticle redness and inflammation, and even infection.

Breakout

Karen never had pimples as a teenager, so it was a shock when she started to break out in her forties. She'd never heard of adult-onset acne. As Karen was in perimenopause stage, hormonal imbalance was a factor, but her frantic lifestyle didn't help. A mother with a full-time career, plus elderly parents in poor health, Karen never found any time for herself to relax, and it showed on her skin.

If you notice an increase or worsening of pimples or acne breakouts when you are going through a stressful time, you're not alone. Recent research has highlighted the link between increased stress levels and increased breakouts in adults. These breakouts most commonly occur on the face, but can also form on the back, neck, chest, or even upper arms. This relationship between stress and pimples has been related to an imbalance and increase in production of certain hormones during stressful periods. People who are acne-prone, or have a history of adolescent acne, may also find that stress can cause a renewed outbreak or exacerbate a current one.

Flare-Up

Harriet had just started university. Coming from a small high school, the switch to a large, intimidating campus felt overwhelming. Halfway into the semester, Harriet started to develop a red, blotchy rash on her back, chest, and neck. Her skin was dry and itchy. The diagnosis: psoriasis, a skin condition that occurs due to stress.

Psoriasis is a condition where areas of skin become inflamed, forming dry, scaly, plaque-like patches of skin. Areas on the arms, hands, elbows, legs, scalp, and feet are most often affected; however, these patches can develop almost anywhere on the body. Psoriasis is often a chronic condition, involving recurrent, persistent flare-ups over the course of a lifetime. It is regarded as an autoimmune condition, with genetic and environmental causes both implicated in its development. While a psoriasis flare-up can be uncomfortable, embarrassing, and stressful in itself, stress has been identified as not only a consequence, but also a trigger and aggravator of the condition. Initial outbreaks of psoriasis have also been associated with stressful life periods, and increases in stress levels appear to be related to the presence and severity of a flare-up.

Your Beauty Mental Health Check

Is stress impacting the way *you* look and feel? The impact of stress can affect you in four different ways: mentally, emotionally, physically, and behaviorally.

Go through the following checklist and note any symptoms that you experience.

Mental (Cognitive) Symptoms:
- Poor concentration
- Memory lapses
- Racing thoughts
- Persistent worry
- Difficulty making decisions and poor judgment

Emotional Symptoms:
- Moodiness—both up and down
- Shortness of temper and irritability
- A sense of being overwhelmed

- Agitation
- Easily angered and intolerant
- Inability to relax

Physical Symptoms:
- Increased aches and pains
- Nausea or dizziness
- Rapid heartbeat
- Irritable bowel syndrome
- Poor sex drive
- Frequent colds and flu

Behavioral Symptoms:
- Increased or reduced appetite
- Needing more or less sleep than usual
- Procrastination
- Increased alcohol, nicotine, or drug use
- Nervous habits—nail biting, pacing, etc.

If you noted five or more of these symptoms, you are likely experiencing negative stress. No matter what age you are, don't wait for the symptoms to appear or get worse before you take action.

Use the mindful beauty treatments in this book to make some positive changes *now*.

Five Pillars of Mindful Beauty

The revolutionary mindful beauty treatments that follow reflect five mindfulness concepts to improve well-being. You will be gently guided to learn, develop, and maintain your skills in these areas. Each mindful beauty treatment utilizes one or more of these life-enhancing concepts:

AWARENESS

Increasing awareness of yourself and your surroundings is a key aspect of mindfulness. You'll learn mindful beauty techniques to develop your attention and engage your senses through exercises such as visualization and focusing, as well as simple breathing and meditation practices. Face and body scanning will increase your consciousness and body responsiveness as well as your felt sense of self. You'll become more mindful of your bodily sensations, thoughts, and feelings, as well as the everyday and natural world around you.

ACCEPTANCE

Accepting ourselves as we are—our bodies, minds, and emotions—is the next step in mindfulness training. Mindful beauty techniques include meditation and mirror work to develop a nonjudgmental stance and become more accepting and approving of how you look. Cognitive training methods will help with negative self-talk and boost your beauty and body esteem. You will develop a life-changing attitude shift toward yourself.

EXERCISE

Mindfulness builds mental muscle. It's a practice that has an initial pay-off and even better long-term benefits, just like going to the gym. Mindful beauty meditations that train your mind go hand in hand with physical training, including better beauty and self-care strategies, on-the-spot stress-reduction tools, affirmations, and bad mood busters that exercise your body and mind.

RELAXATION

Once you're mindful of your physical, mental, and emotional state, it's easier to let go. Mindful beauty relaxation techniques include stress-reduction practices, face and body muscle relaxation methods, tools to release physical and mental tension, as well as ways to revive beauty and self-care rituals that have an added benefit when carried out in a more mindful way. You'll soon feel more calm and beautiful.

LOVING-KINDNESS

Loving-kindness is both a result and practice of mindfulness. Mindful beauty techniques include contemplation and consciousness-raising that increase your self-care and compassion, and bring joy and gentleness into your everyday beauty routines. You'll learn how to practice many acts of kindness toward yourself and see who you are with a more loving gaze.

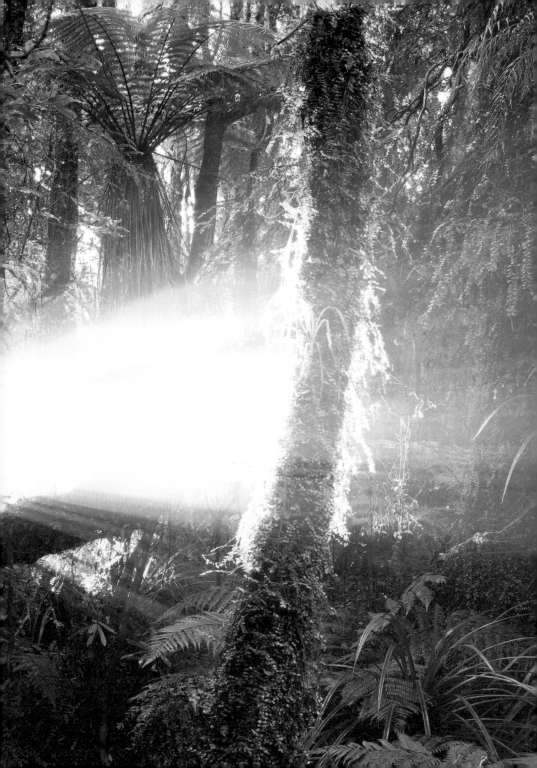

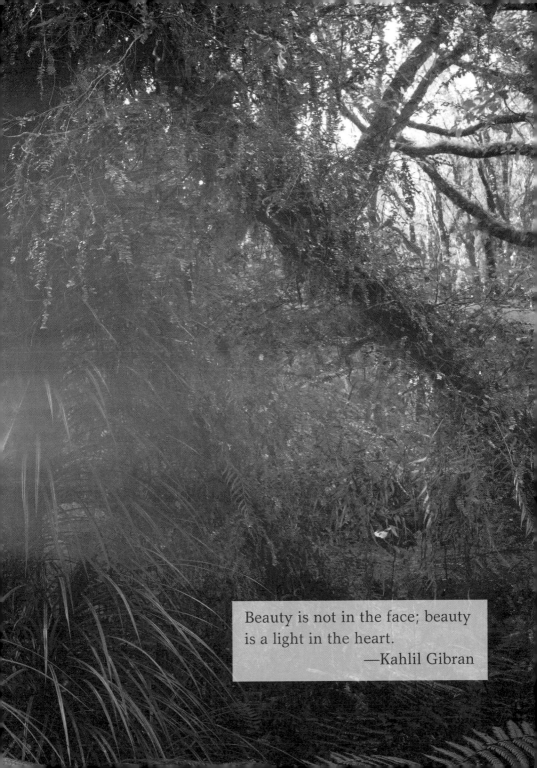

Beauty is not in the face; beauty
is a light in the heart.
—Kahlil Gibran

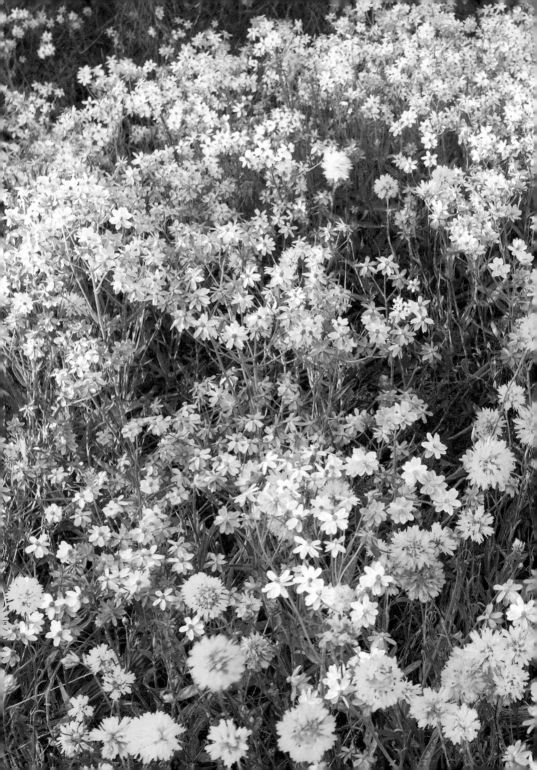

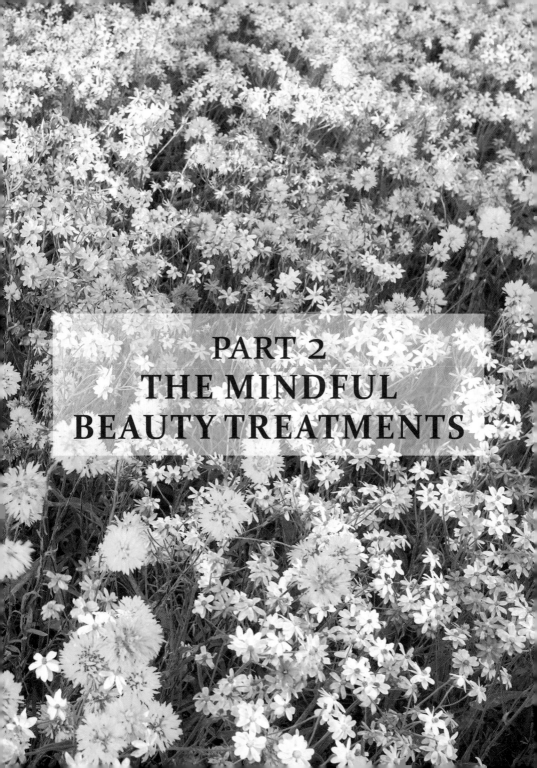

PART 2
THE MINDFUL
BEAUTY TREATMENTS

1 Where You Dwell: Making Space for Mindful Beauty

Where do you put on your makeup? Where do you cleanse your skin or brush your hair? In the bathroom, in the bedroom, in the kitchen, in the car, in bed, on the run?

Consider the physical space you make for yourself and this aspect of your self-care. Notice if it is clean or cluttered, ordered or in disarray.

Make no judgment about your self-care space at this time. Simply notice and accept it. Paying attention is the first step. As you practice mindful beauty, you'll make changes to your physical surroundings that will emerge spontaneously and joyfully. You'll want to give yourself the space and time you deserve. Be prepared to dwell in a different beauty space as you become more acquainted with mindful beauty.

Where you dwell also applies to your mental and emotional state. Dwelling on things, our problems, worries, or flaws, is also known as rumination. When we get hooked into repetitive, damaging thoughts, it's as if we live in a place we can't escape. Our thoughts become habitual, a grind that wears us down. Mindfulness is like a breath of fresh air; it throws open the window and lets in the light. The more you practice mindful beauty, the more you'll experience a lightening of your mental state. You'll know how to flip the switch. You won't dwell in negativity so much anymore. You'll keep your mental space airy and light. Mindful beauty techniques will especially help you in the area of self-care, beauty, and body esteem, but you can expect these techniques to bring relief and to enhance pleasure in other areas of your life as well.

Your emotions too, won't feel so heavy and burdensome. Mindfulness teaches us that any time we choose we can vacate rooms where we don't want to stay. It doesn't mean those dark corners no longer exist, but we can close the door on them, and step into the light. Mindful beauty helps you access brighter emotional dimensions and more positive places to be. Your preferences for these places of health and beauty will lead you to linger there more and more, as you become more aware and adept at accessing them.

Your body is also your dwelling place. As you proceed through the mindful beauty process, you'll become tuned into the mind-body connection more powerfully. Your body will give you clues to your feelings in ways you never noticed before. Vice-versa, you'll recognize where your emotions manifest in your body, and you'll be able to soothe and de-stress those areas before they settle into tension or pain, before they become etched into your skin. You'll diagnose body sensations with more ease and awareness and know how to address them instantly.

Fresh-Faced: Start with a Beginner's Mind
This is a short and simple exercise to begin. You can practice it whenever you start a self-care routine.

One of the key concepts in mindfulness is to start with a beginner's mind. This means putting away preconceived ideas of how things are or how they ought to be.

Let's start with your face. Remove all makeup. Pull back long hair from your face in a simple ponytail (not too tight). Stand in front of a mirror and take a fresh look at you. Imagine you are meeting this person for the first time. How does she look? What color and texture is her hair? Is it dark, fair, curly, wavy, or straight? Describe it aloud. What shape is her face: oval, rectangular, round? What color are her eyes: blue, green, gray, brown, hazel? Try describing the subtleties in shade. What shape are her eyebrows? Are they fine or thick, arched or winged? Now her nose. Is it long, short, aquiline, snub, freckled? What about her skin? Describe her complexion. Now her lips. What color is her natural lip tone? Is her chin firm or full? If a judgment or emotion comes up, this is common. We are used to examining ourselves in a judgmental or critical way. Try to catch yourself in the act, perhaps labeling your face shape as too round, or your lips too thin. Just acknowledge these thoughts, then shift your awareness back to the feature you are focusing on.

Jon Kabat-Zinn suggests that we regularly remind ourselves "this is it." For mindful beauty, we can regularly remind ourselves "this is me."

Take a look at this face as a whole. This is you *now*. Forget the you of the past. Forget the future you. This is how you look today, in the present moment.

Say hello to you.

Bring Some "Beautility" to Your Self-Care Space: Bell, Book, and Candle

In the nineteenth century, the word *beautility* was coined by Ada Louise Huxtable, an American architectural critic. The word aimed to capture the qualities of space and design that are conducive to both beauty and usefulness.

You can prepare your physical dwelling space for a mindful change by bringing some *beautility* to your self-care surroundings.

1. *Light a candle.* Candles have long been a way to bring us into a more peaceful and reflective state of mind, as well as beautifying

our surroundings. Select a candle in a color or aroma that you find especially appealing. Light the candle before your beauty routine begins, and blow it out when your routine is complete.

2. *Ring a bell*. In many mindfulness and meditation practices, a gong or bell is rung at the beginning and end of a session. Add a small bell to your bathroom counter or dressing table. Ring the bell once before you begin any beauty treatment or self-care routine and once again at the end to remind you to stay mindful during the process.

3. *Attend to your posture*. As well as paying attention to what is around you, pay attention to your body's architecture. Adopt the classic meditation pose when you complete a beauty task. This is also known as a mindful attitude, capturing both our body and mind. Stand or sit with a relaxed but upright posture, with your back and neck straight. Place equal weight on both feet. Let your arms and shoulders be relaxed as you undertake your beauty routine.

4. Keep your book of mindful beauty close by.

Dwell in beauty. Dwell in harmony. Dwell in well-being.

Quick Lift: See Small Beauties

Wherever you are right now, take a moment to study your surroundings and notice something beautiful. It might be a plant or flower, a person, an ornament, or an artifact. It might be something on your desk, on the street, in a shop window, or through your window. Whatever you alight upon, give it your full attention. Appreciate its beauty. As you practice this more and more, you'll find that you notice more small beauties in the world around you. Your awareness of beauty will increase and multiply. The more you practice mindful beauty, the more beautiful your life will become. Even things you never thought beautiful before will gain beauty in your eyes. Your perception will expand to encompass many forms of beauty. And that includes you.

The Secrets of Mindful Beauty

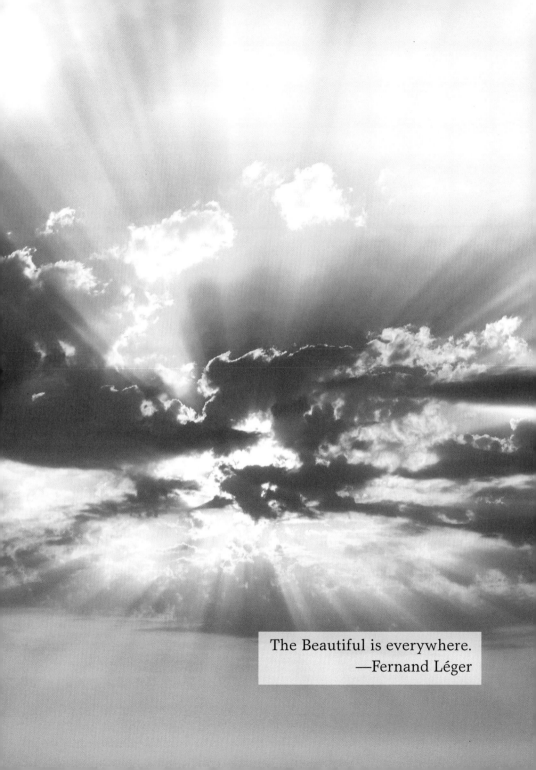

The Beautiful is everywhere.
—Fernand Léger

2 Oxygenate Your Skin: Breathe Your Way to a Clear Complexion

Mindfulness is beautifully simple.

You don't have to know a lot about mindfulness or meditation to gain the benefits of mindful beauty. All it takes to start is a breath of fresh air.

As a self-awareness skill, mindfulness focuses on sensation, experiencing the present moment, and accepting things in a nonjudgmental way. Practicing mindfulness is valuable in our everyday lives and can assist in decreasing overall stress and worry. Once you've tried it, you can bring it into other areas of your life. You will be able to focus on the here and now, instead of worrying about the future or ruminating on the past. This can seem like a lot to bring together all at once, but there is an easy way to center yourself and find the still point within. A useful anchor for bringing yourself into the present moment is your breath.

Mindful breathing has a dual benefit: it helps treat anxiety and boosts your skin cells. It will help you stay refreshed and fight fatigue. There are many expensive salon treatments that add some extra oxygen to your skin. Consider improving your own breathing technique first. With this mindful breathing method, you can do it yourself for free.

Our breathing is closely connected to our anxiety and stress levels. Hyperventilation can be responsible for the feelings of panic or acute anxiety that some people experience. Hyperventilation is characterized by rapid, shallow, uneven breaths and can lead to a faster heart rate, tingling sensations in the body, chest pains, and dizziness. One way to address this problem is to alter your breathing when these signs emerge.

Breathing exercises can also be helpful for people with high levels of general stress and worry. Findings suggest that a lot of people "under-breathe," only taking shallow, superficial breaths. This can lead to headaches, dizziness, and even feelings of nausea. Next time you feel anxious, turn your attention to your breathing. You may be breathing faster and in a more shallow way than normal. You may even be holding your breath.

Mindful breathing can also help with freak-out face. One of the poor thinking traps many anxiety-prone people fall into is disaster thinking and catastrophizing. This line of thinking occurs when certain events are viewed from an extreme frame of mind, which can lead to disaster for our faces and bodies. Consider how you look when you're freaked out. Aaagh! If our body is regularly in this state, it can become exhausting, with damaging effects on our appearance. With mindful breathing, the uncomfortable physiological responses in your body can be reduced. Say good-bye to your freak-out face and say hello to the source of calm within.

Breathe into Beauty Exercise

This easy exercise can be used to practice better breathing habits. Use it every time you are about to begin an element of your beauty routine or self-care. Try it for the first time when you are feeling relatively relaxed. It can be practiced standing or sitting.

Place your hand on your diaphragm. Breathe in through your nose, counting to three. Try to draw your breath deep into your belly, toward your hand. Hold your breath in for a further two counts and release, breathing out through your mouth. Repeat this ten times, concentrating on drawing your breath downward.

By incorporating mindful breathing into your regular beauty routine, you will become more adept at this simple technique. Next time you are feeling stressed, anxious, or panicked, try to follow this pattern of mindful breathing. Slow, even breathing is incompatible with panicky feelings, like heart palpitations and dizziness. Mindfully breathe yourself back to beauty.

Finding Your Breath Home Base

This next exercise will take you even deeper into your breathing.

Sit in a comfortable, quiet place. Take up your meditation posture, keeping your spine straight. Don't slouch or curl your body.

Gently close your eyes and begin to focus on your breathing. We're going to explore different breath sites in your body to find your breath home base.

Direct your attention to the tip of your nose. Feel the breath going in and out. Notice the sensation. Explore how it feels. Rest your attention in that part of your body. Breathe in and out of your nose a few times.

Now direct your attention to your mouth. Open it slightly. Feel the breath going in and out. Notice the sensation, pleasant or unpleasant, accepting what is there. Does it make a sound? Explore how it feels. Rest your attention in that part of your body. Breathe in and out of your mouth.

Direct your attention to your throat. Can you feel the breath moving in your throat? Notice the sensation, pleasant or unpleasant, accepting what is there. Explore how it feels. Does it feel warm or cool? Focus your attention in that part of your body. Breathe in and out a few times, attending to the air moving at the back of your throat.

Direct your attention to your chest. Can you feel the breath in your chest? Notice the sensation, pleasant or unpleasant, accepting what is there. Notice your chest rising and falling. Explore how it feels. Place your hand on your chest if it helps. Find the place in your chest where you notice the breath most. Rest your attention in that part of your body. Breathe in and out a few times, attending to the air moving in your chest.

Direct your attention to your diaphragm. Can you feel the breath reaching your diaphragm? Perhaps you are noticing the movement of your body as the breath rises and falls. Explore how it feels. Notice the sensation, pleasant or unpleasant, accepting what is there, perhaps placing your hand just below your rib cage if it helps. Rest your attention in that part of your body. Breathe in and out a few times, keeping your focus on your diaphragm.

Now direct your attention to your lower belly. Can you feel the breath in your belly? Notice the sensation, pleasant or unpleasant, accepting what is there. Notice your belly rising and falling. Explore how it feels. Place your hand on your belly if it helps. Find the place where you notice the breath most. Rest your attention in that part of your body. Breathe in and out a few times, focusing on your belly.

Gently open your eyes.

In what area of the body did you experience your breath most? Nose, mouth, throat, chest, diaphragm, or belly? This is your breath home base.

It may take a few meditative explorations to find your breath home base. Try it as many times as you like. Explore. You can also try this meditation lying down or standing. This will help you access your true breath home base.

When you know your breath home base, it will become a place of familiarity, rest, and refuge for you. Whenever you do a breath meditation, you can gently take your attention to your home base.

Finding the Gap

Mindfulness teaches us to look for the gap—the silent spaces in our consciousness that aren't full of self-talk and busyness in our brains. Our beauty routines are wonderful points each day to find a welcome gap in our lives. When we look into the mirror, or practice some self-care, it reminds us that we have a body. We're not just a busy brain. Each time we look at ourselves we have the gift of a moment to take some space and time, to remind ourselves that we can take a break and have a rest, even for a few seconds. Instead of viewing our beauty rituals and routines as yet another task to be rushed through, we can reframe them as a refreshing, restful gap.

Take Time to Breathe Exercise

Start with your morning routine. This is often an opportunity for the first gap at the start of your day. Take a moment to recognize this gap when you first look in the mirror, before you wash your face, style your hair, or begin to apply makeup.

Stop. Close your eyes. Breathe. Just three times. In. Out. In. Out. In. Out. Just breathe and be still, even if it is only for a few seconds. Find that moment of inner silence. The gap will grow.

Continue to give yourself these beautiful moments throughout the day. Find the gap when you look at yourself in the mirror at any other time of the day, to touch up your makeup, to check your teeth after a meal, to wash your hands in the restroom. (It's called a restroom for a reason, remember?) Remind yourself: this is a welcome gap in my day. Close your eyes and breathe in and out three times. Luxuriate in the space of a moment's pause.

In the evening, before removing your makeup or cleaning your teeth, stop. Pause. Close your eyes and take three deep breaths.

As you find the gaps in this simple way, you'll discover it has a timeless quality. When you return to the time-bound world, life will seem slower and much less hurried. You'll instantly look calmer and more peaceful too.

When you become more practiced in deep breathing, you may notice that you observe a gap between your breaths. Experts in meditation and yoga can extend this gap between breaths, creating a portal to deep awareness. Notice if the gaps between your breath grow as you go deeper into mindful beauty.

Seek the spaces of peace and silence that are most precious. Your daily beauty routines are the places you will find these moments—and find yourself again.

Quick Lift: Just Add Water

Follow your breathing exercise with a refreshing glass of water. H_2O is a great way to improve your skin tone by keeping it hydrated. Double the amount of water you drink and take another slow lung full of air when you've emptied the glass. Appreciate the refreshing beauty of your breath.

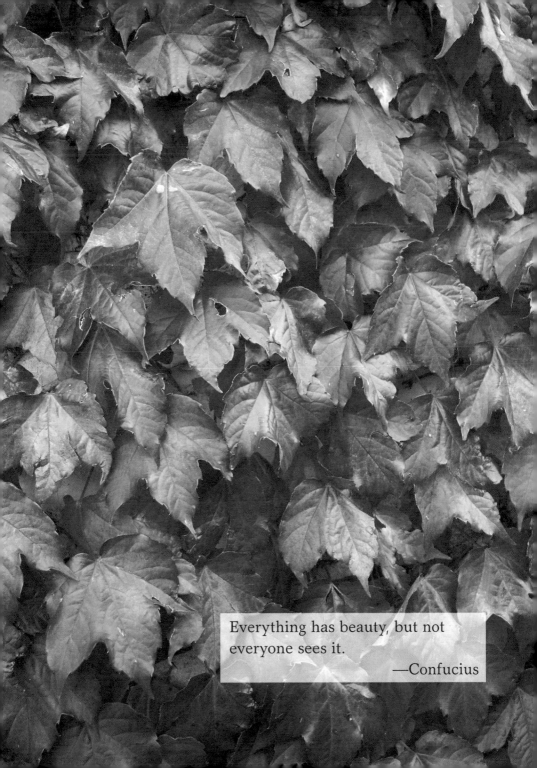

Everything has beauty, but not everyone sees it.

—Confucius

3. Makeup with Mindfulness: Refocus Your Makeup and Skin Routine

Salve for Your Soul

Paying attention to your own touch is beneficial whenever you apply any makeup, lotion, cream, or oil to your skin.

In the past, applying ointments and salves was considered a spiritual practice. A salve was a soft healing ointment that was also a spiritual remedy. The word *salven* (linked to salvation) means to heal or treat spiritually. It was connected to the practice of applying salves and balms to our skin with the utmost sanctity and respect.

Bringing back this sense of respect and sacredness to our beauty routines is part of mindful beauty. In the Buddhist mindfulness tradition, seeing the holiness of the everyday, appreciating the wholeness of each moment, is an essential element of the practice. It's part of other spiritual traditions too. Holiness, wholeness, and healing are interconnected—mind, body, spirit. Engaging the spiritual remedy of our own healing touch is how we can soothe our skin . . . and ourselves.

Makeup with Mindfulness

How you apply your makeup is just as important as what you apply. If you're treating yourself and your skin harshly, it's going to show.

No more rushing through your skin care routine, slapping on some makeup, removing your mascara with angry strokes, or glaring at yourself in the mirror each morning. This unique makeup method provides a simple way to practice mindfulness, teaching you how to focus on your face in the way you deserve.

Applying and removing makeup is one area in our lives that often becomes automatic. It's possible to miss the signs that we might be applying makeup incorrectly, or damaging our skin as we remove it. Using mindfulness is a great way to bring focus back to the present, and reexamine how we go about our automatic beauty routines.

Under Pressure

You can start to increase your mind-body awareness by considering the pressure you put yourself under whenever you apply makeup or a skin care product. Take a moment to consider it when you next apply a product with your fingers. Notice if the pressure is right for you. How would you describe the level of pressure: soft, gentle, soothing, firm, medium, brisk, hard, heavy, or painful? Notice if you are light-fingered or heavy-handed. If the pressure isn't right for you, adjust it. It might take a few times to relearn with your fingers and a few fine adjustments. Allow time to learn a new habit. Be mindful whenever you apply pressure.

Applying Makeup Mindfully Exercise

- Begin in front of your bathroom mirror or dressing table, with all your makeup at hand. Allow some extra time for your routine. Try to keep distractions to a minimum (no music or TV in the background).
- Start your makeup routine, paying attention to each step you take. Go slowly. If your attention wanders, bring it back to your routine.

- Apply a soothing moisturizer. Think about how the moisturizer feels on your skin when it is applied and how it smells. Look at your reflection as you apply it, focusing on how you are applying it to your skin; are you rubbing it in harshly, or are you patting it on smoothly? Look at the facial expressions you make, are you frowning, crinkling up your eyes? Be gentle.
- Apply foundation and blush. Again, consider how it feels on your skin when applied. Inhale the scent, and appreciate the color and texture whether it's a cream, a mousse, or a lotion, and how it feels. Notice if it matches your skin. Observe what you're covering up, and what you're revealing. Look at your reflection, focusing on how you are applying it to your skin. Do you smooth it in with your fingers, or are you pressing down too firmly? If you use a brush, do the bristles hurt you, or are you using light strokes?
- Apply your eye makeup. Really take in the color of your eyes. Enjoy the different shades of eye shadows, liners, and mascara you have to choose from. What emotions do the colors evoke in you? When you apply your eye makeup, notice the expressions you make, are you crinkling up your eyes? Relax your delicate eye area.
- Apply lipstick or lip balm. Consider the colors you choose, as well as the texture. What does it smell like? What's the flavor? When you apply it, are you puckering up your mouth, creating lines, or are you forming a relaxed oval? Smile at yourself when you're done.
- Complete this exercise for each makeup step. You may include other steps as needed. Focus on the sensations you experience during your routine, what you see, smell, and feel.

Mindfulness may sound simple, but you'll notice great results. Not only will you have applied your makeup more carefully, but you will have also reduced your stress by slowing yourself down and focusing on the present, rather than your internal processes and thoughts. It's a great way to start the day.

Removing Makeup Mindfully Exercise

Mindfulness can also be used when removing makeup. Placing attention on how we remove our makeup, and how our skin feels when we do, can also help us identify any rough treatment our skin might be receiving. Notice if your skin is smarting or stinging after you have washed your face. The delicate skin around your eyes may be burning slightly. Perhaps you are removing your foundation too harshly, or perhaps the toner you are using is too abrasive. Take the time to reflect on treating yourself gently.

A Fresh Take on Beauty Products

There are so many beauty products available, all of which seem to offer us the "miracle fix." However, can we really be sure that they do what they promise? Ultimately, the answer is no. Whether we think we have found THE product, or whether we are feeling as though we have been conned once again, there is a new way we can consider the time and money we invest in our cosmetics and products, which is to enjoy the *experience* of them. Rather than choosing something because you think it is the best, choose something because you like it. Take time to connect to the experience of selecting and buying a product. Do you like how it smells? Does it come in a beautiful bottle? When you use it, how does it make you feel? Does it make you notice the scent of roses all day? Does it feel smooth and silky to apply? Does it fill your bathroom with a delightful aroma? Notice how you feel when you apply the product. Do you feel different? Do you feel more confident with a specific shade of lipstick, or a particular perfume? All of these are valid reasons to invest in these products, because it becomes about investing in you.

Replenishing Your Beauty Supplies Exercise

When you are replenishing your beauty supplies, mindfulness can help with your purchasing choices by increasing your awareness of the sensations and emotions being supplied to you in that moment.

Before you purchase a beauty product, check the following.

1. **Body sensations**—Is your body relaxed and at ease? Is there any tension in your body?
2. **Emotions**—What feelings are evoked by your intended purchase? Notice whether you label these positive, neutral, or negative.

If you experience any discomfort, reconsider your purchase or explore the reason why. If you feel comfortable, proceed and take home beauty products that fully supply you.

Makeup Extras

- Smile at yourself whenever you apply makeup. Beam yourself some approval.
- Greet your reflection with "You look fantastic!" or "Absolutely fabulous!"
- Attach a sticker to the corner of your mirror (such as a flower or another symbol that is special to you) as a mindfulness reminder.
- Step into the light. Check your makeup in some natural daylight. Appreciate the beauty around you and in you.

Quick Lift: Make Up Your Mind

Mindful beauty is a choice. It's a decision you make to attend to yourself and what is around you, rather than remain on automatic. It isn't always easy, but it becomes easier once you make up your mind to be mindful. Check in with yourself and focus on being rather than doing. Keep making that decision, moment by moment.

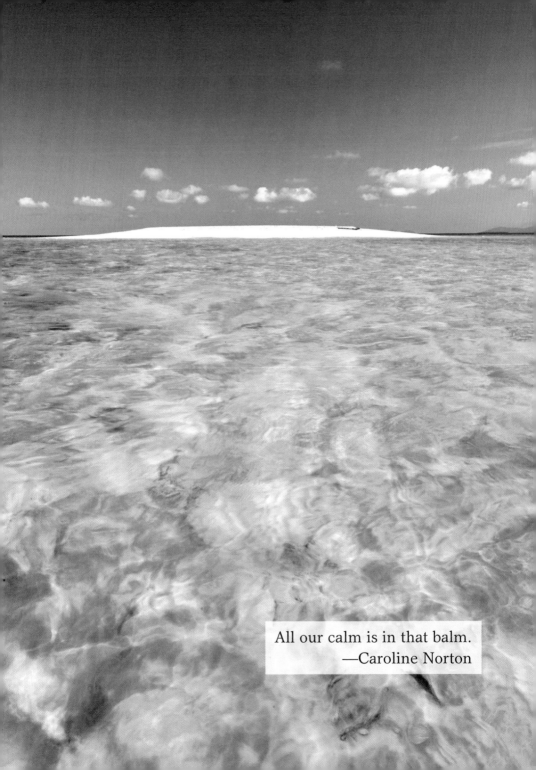

All our calm is in that balm.
—Caroline Norton

4 Mirror a Loving Gaze: Developing Positive Regard

What we see in our minds is reflected on our faces. If we want to reflect beauty outwardly, we need to be able to see it within.

Psychologists refer to a concept called unconditional positive regard. This comes from the humanistic psychological tradition of client-centered therapy, developed in the 1970s by Carl Rogers. Unconditional positive regard means to accept other people and view them with respect, just as they are. Like mindfulness, the approach avoids judgment and evaluation.

When we regard another person, we look up to them. To hold someone in high regard is to esteem them, to hold them above others, not putting them on a pedestal, or insisting they are superior, but to really value them. Regard is when we see and are seen for who we really are.

Regard has an older, deeper meaning. It means consideration, paying attention to. It can also invoke an aspect, an appearance, a look. It means to take notice of, look at, to heed, or to watch. It also invokes a quality of looking, to view with esteem, with affection, or with kindly feeling.

Increasing your positive self-regard takes practice. You can practice it every time you look in the mirror by accepting and being aware of what you see. Take notice of any judgments that come when you regard yourself, without falling into the trap of judging yourself for being judgmental! The following techniques will help you build up some positive self-regard.

Facial Scanning: Identifying Trouble Spots

Without being aware of it, many of us create tension and trouble spots in our faces and bodies. We all have areas where we hold tension, and it shows up on the surface of our skin sooner or later unless we practice some preventative methods.

Facial and body scanning is a relaxation technique. It is also a mindfulness strategy that helps us connect and become aware of our bodies and ourselves in the present moment. Relaxation techniques are an important and effective way of reducing the physical signs and symptoms of anxiety and stress. Sometimes the sensations associated with anxiety are uncomfortable or painful. By learning how to address the physical symptoms, we can help reduce our anxiety levels. It's a great way to bring awareness to any anxiety or tension that might be held in your face, neck, and shoulders. Mindful facial and body scanning can be used whenever feelings of tension arise.

Facial Scanning Exercise

- Begin by sitting or lying down somewhere comfortable and quiet. Close your eyes and start to focus on your breathing, inhaling slowly and deeply, and then exhaling. Focus on your breathing for five more breaths.
- Turn your focus to your forehead and temples. Is your brow smooth, or is it tightened? Allow all the muscles in your forehead to relax.
- Turn your attention to your eye area. Think about how your eyes feel, are you squeezing them shut or are they gently closed? Soften any muscle tension you may feel around your eyes as you continue to breathe slowly.

- Focus on your jaw. Are you clenching your teeth together? Allow your teeth to separate slightly.
- Now focus on your mouth and lips. Is your mouth pursed, or are your lips pressed together? Soften any tense muscles and continue breathing deeply and slowly.
- Move your attention to your neck. Is your head hanging forward, or are you holding it at an angle? Try lifting your head up and tipping it back, allowing your neck to lengthen.
- Focus on your shoulders and upper back. Do you notice any strain or tension across your shoulders and upper back? Are you holding your shoulders rigidly? Try relaxing and lowering your shoulders a little.
- Finish by shifting your focus back to your breathing, keeping your breaths slow and deep.

Body Scanning Extension:
- Extend this scanning technique across your whole body, starting at your head and finishing at your toes. It is best to try this lying down. This exercise can help you identify other areas of your body where you might habitually hold tension, while also achieving a completely relaxed state.

Regular practice of facial and body scanning can assist you in reducing overall stress and tension levels. What's more, it will alert you to the areas in your body where you hold on to anxiety. Identify your trouble spots, and then practice face and body scanning to release them. While doing these exercises, remember that it's normal to get distracted by thoughts. The trick is then to bring your attention back to your face and body.

Contemplation: Cultivating a Loving Gaze
Contemplation is a practice similar to meditation, although there are some differences. Meditation requires some focus; we concentrate on

our breath, on a mantra or prayer, or perhaps a particular picture or symbol. In contrast, contemplation lets our thoughts roam free. It means to "survey with the eyes or the mind." The word contemplate comes from the Latin *contemplari* which was linked to the word *templum* (temple), in which an oracle resided. Contemplation accesses the temple of your mind through the temple of your body.

Contemplation is a useful complement to mindfulness. You may appear to be doing nothing, when, in fact, you're doing a lot. While it may appear to be no more than daydreaming, it's actually a way of widening your eyes to what you see. In Sanskrit, this is known as dharma: opening ourselves to the world and what we experience.

Poets and philosophers have always valued contemplation, especially contemplation of the natural world. For example, William Wordsworth, who "wandered lonely as a cloud" and famously reflected on the beauty of daffodils, writes about contemplation in his poem, "The Prelude":

When Contemplation, like the night-calm felt
Through earth and sky, spreads widely, and sends deep
Into the soul its tranquillising power,

Contemplation has also been called "the loving gaze." All too often, the gaze we turn upon ourselves is anything but loving. It can be harsh and judgmental. Unfortunately, a harsh gaze can come from the world around us and become how we see ourselves. In the seventies, feminists referred to what they called "the male gaze." This gaze, from the masculine perspective, objectified women. It was argued that many girls and women internalized this perspective, viewing themselves as objects to be looked at, rather than experiencing their own point of view. There's also a female gaze, which gives other women the once-over in a way that can be competitive, scrutinizing, or spiteful. We may also have experienced a critical gaze when we were growing up, perhaps at school or from a family member. Perhaps we still hear harsh comments from others or ourselves. No wonder it's so hard to look at ourselves with loving-kindness. But we can learn to see clearly again.

Contemplari: *Reflective Visualization Exercise*

Try this visualization technique. This is a creative process you can carry out as often as you wish.

You can stand, sit, or lie down for this exercise. Close your eyes. Allow ten to twenty minutes. Bring to your mind the most beautiful place you have ever seen. It might be somewhere you visited or a place you saw in a movie or on TV. It might be mountains, woods, the beach, a starry sky, or a city skyline. It might be far away or it may be near home. Visit this place in your mind.

Allow yourself to fully experience this place. Look around, breathe the air. Engage all of your senses. See all that is around you with your eyes and your mind by cultivating a state of calm and relaxed receptivity. Glance in front of you, sideways, look over your shoulder. Gaze around, breathe the air. Stop and stare. Engage all your senses—take note of what you see, smell, hear, and touch. Pay attention to every detail, but without strain. Stand back and take in the whole. Relax. Contemplate your surroundings for as long as you like; let its beauty become part of you.

In your mind, change the visual. Picture you are face to face with someone you love who is giving you a beautiful smile. Who is that person? Notice the feelings your body is having in response to this image. In your mind, visit with them for as long as you like. Let the love you share become part of you.

Change the visual again and picture your own face. Contemplate your face just as you did in the location you thought of previously and the face of a person you love. Can you continue to feel that beauty and love? Can you keep bringing it to you? Feel it in your heart, the loving-kindness spreading through your body.

Now, open your eyes. Go to a mirror. Allow the beauty of your contemplations to remain expressed in your eyes, mind, face, and body. Let your loving gaze include you.

Next time you go somewhere or see something beautiful, contemplate it. Create a picture in your mind for further contemplation. You can also use your contemplative image for visualization. There's no limit to the beauty you can contemplate outside and inside you. It is always accessible, always there. You are part of the world's beauty. It is part of you.

Quick Lift: Mindful Check-In

Sometimes there are certain places or situations that contribute to our level of worry, stress, and negativity. Do you fall asleep with a frown on your face? Do you wait at traffic lights with a furrowed brow and gritted teeth? Try putting a visual reminder in the places where worry and stress hit you the most, like your car, your bedside table, or your desk at work. It could be something like a sticker, a plastic flower, even a Post-it note. Every time you see it, it will serve as a reminder to do a mindful check-in and a quick face and body scan: are you frowning? Clenching your jaw? Let that tension go.

The Secrets of Mindful Beauty

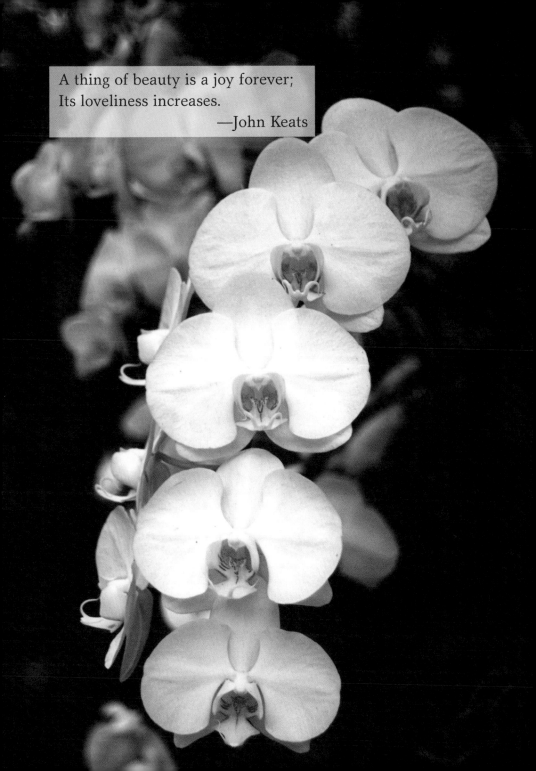

A thing of beauty is a joy forever;
Its loveliness increases.
—John Keats

5 Beauty in a Bottle: Appreciating Cosmetic Artistry

Top beauty brands employ some of the best artists and designers in the world. An enjoyable mindful beauty technique is to become more aware and appreciative of your cosmetics in a new way, by noticing their beautiful containers. From supermarket buys to exclusive brands, they are individual works of art and design. Each cosmetic container, if you look closely, is a work of art, an expression of creativity that meets the mindful beauty criteria of *beautility:* being both beautiful and useful.

Appreciation of Cosmetic Art

Follow these simple steps to become more mindful of the cosmetic artistry around you.

Hold. Pick up a cosmetic container. It can be a perfume bottle, a skin care product, a hair product, or a makeup container, anything from eye makeup to lipstick. Hold it in the palm of your hand.

Observe. Take your time to focus on the container with attention and care. Imagine it's the first time you have ever seen this product. With your eyes, explore and examine it. Hold it up to the light or a window to see it better. Notice where light shines on it, its shape, color, and symmetry.

Touch. Pass the container from one hand to the other. Examine its size and shape. Notice if it fits comfortably in your hand. Explore its silhouette, its corners, whether it is flat-sided or multidimensional. Try this with your eyes closed to enhance your sense of touch.

Hear. Does the product make a sound? Does it open with a click or close with a snap? What can you hear if you gently shake the container? Does the lid come off with a pop?

Smell. Notice if the product has a scent. You may be able to smell the fragrance even when the container is closed. Inhale. Take in the fragrance. Open the container and inhale again.

Place. Now, place the container on your dressing table or bathroom counter. Notice where you placed it, how it sits. Review it as part of your cosmetic collection. Note its proportions, large or small, and how it is enhanced by what is around it.

Use this mindfulness procedure to explore your cosmetics and the beauty of their individual containers, as well as how they appear as a group. You can use it as a slow-down technique, to avoid rushing through your beauty routine. By selecting one container at a time, you'll use your cosmetics with more care and display them more attractively as well. Even better, you'll slow down and enjoy them more.

Bottled Beauty

- Clean the outer cases of your cosmetics. Make them shine.
- Display your cosmetics on a shelf.
- Buy a beauty product for the pure pleasure of its aesthetic appearance.
- Select your most beautiful cosmetic. Give it pride of place.
- Color-code your cosmetics.
- Sort your cosmetics according to size or shape.

- Place your cosmetics in front of a mirror or on a mirror to increase their reflection.
- Collect perfume bottles.
- Decant cosmetics into containers, jars, and bottles you like. Seek out glass, plastic, or vintage.
- Hunt for vintage cosmetic cases, such as powder pots, vanity boxes, and compacts.
- Seek out an old dressing table set to contain your cosmetics.

Visit a Cosmetic Gallery

Make a visit to the cosmetic area of a department store or beauty supply store. These glittering emporiums are full of fabulous works of art.

Behave as if you are visiting a gallery or museum. Look at all the different displays and art collections. Lean in to examine a particular piece. Take your time to wander and wonder. Notice what is around you. Indulge your senses. Engage your sight and inhale the scents. Touch the different containers, jars, and bottles. Hold them in your hands. Examine their intricacies and details. Stand back and admire whole displays. Explore your artistic preferences and identify your favorite styles and designs. Appreciate the artful production of beauty.

The Present Moment: Your Free Gifts

Tote bags, cosmetic purses, makeup bags, miniature scents and lotions, travel-size skin care products, tiny eye shadow palettes, and mini tubes of lipstick—who doesn't love a free gift?

Once or twice a year, many cosmetic companies give away a clutch of sample-size gifts with the purchase of their products. These gifts introduce us to new products, remind us of old favorites, and feature new colors of the season.

It was Estée Lauder who first invented the gift-with-purchase concept in the fifties, and it has been enjoyed ever since. It isn't only a material pleasure. Giving and receiving gifts triggers happiness in our brains, boosting our health and well-being.

Mindful beauty offers us free gifts too, through present moment awareness. You can make the most of being here right now, by appreciating what is freely given to you.

Unwrap your free gifts:
- the gift of air
- the gift of light
- the gift of safety
- the gift of health
- the gift of a heartbeat
- the gift of eyesight
- the gift of hearing
- the gift of taste
- the gift of scent
- the gift of touch
- the gift of consciousness
- the gift of yourself

What else is in your gift bag? The act of noticing and appreciating will give you that sense of contentment and delight. You can also freely give to others.

Give away:
- the gift of a smile
- the gift of attention
- the gift of acceptance
- the gift of kindness
- the gift of laughter
- the gift of gentleness
- the gift of compassion

Appreciate and bestow simple gifts upon yourself and others. At any time during the day, gift yourself the present moment. Stop and notice what you're freely given.

Quick Lift: Choose a Mindful Beauty Mascot

A mascot is a personal good luck charm. It's a person, animal, or thing used to summon good fortune. The word mascot originally came from *masca*, an Old French word for witch, and the good luck pieces they carried. *Masca* also meant mask, and is related to the word *mascara*. Old Latin documents sometimes referred to groups of witches as *mascara*.

Choose a mindful beauty mascot. Make it small enough to keep in your cosmetic bag, or select a mascot to ornament your dressing table or bathroom counter, along with your mascara. Let it be a talisman to remind you to stay mindful, and may it accompany you with good luck. You're not alone on your mindful beauty journey.

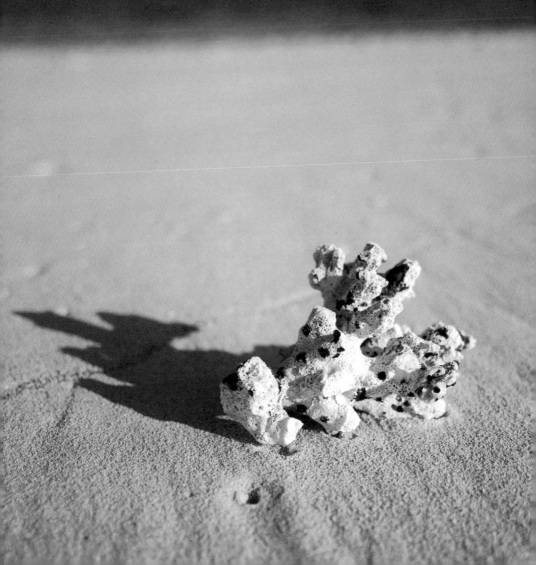

Take your delight in momentariness.
—Robert Graves

6
Clear Cosmetic Clutter: Clarify Your Mind

Clear cosmetic clutter the mindful beauty way. Mindfulness is not only an excellent mental technique to help you focus and relax, it also has a practical application. With mindfulness, you can clean your bathroom cabinets and sink tops, your dressing table drawers and surfaces, and get rid of some problematic attitudes too.

Decluttering Cosmetics Exercise

For this technique choose a time when you are not rushed or stressed. Allow plenty of time to enjoy the task. Make sure you have a trash can nearby and some cleaning products at hand.

Start by examining each of the beauty products you possess. As you pick up each one, ask yourself:

- When did I buy this? Was it weeks, months, or years ago?
- Why did I buy it? What prompted me? What mood was I in?
- How much did it cost? Did I get value for my money or is it over-rated?
- What did I expect it to do? Did it perform?
- Do I waste it? Is it half-used?
- Is it past its expiration date?

Pay special attention to the emotions the beauty products and these questions arise in you. They may be positive or negative. Don't be surprised if they provoke feelings and insights you don't expect. Try to remain nonjudgmental, just notice the thoughts and feelings as they arise.

As you continue to clear the clutter, consider the following:

- Do you have many products? What prompts you to buy them?
- Do you have few? Do you deprive yourself of items you need?
- Do you have multiple products that are meant to do the same thing? Is it an area of concern or an obsession?

Asking these questions will help you clear out the physical clutter and clarify your mental state. Be calm and honest with yourself. Throw away the items you don't need or want, especially if they are past their use by date. Throw away some outdated attitudes too. You don't need them anymore.

Scrub the surfaces and wipe clean all the jars, bottles, and containers. Restock your cosmetic cabinet with the items you have retained: the ones you use and like. You don't need more or less than that.

Continue to clear out your cosmetics on a regular basis and you'll begin to buy them more mindfully as well. You won't double up on extras you already own or haven't used up yet. You won't buy more than you can afford or waste your money. Clear the cosmetic clutter, clean up the money worries, clarify your mind, and you'll have a fresh, clear complexion too.

Cleansing Self-Care
As you go further with mindful beauty, you may notice that you instinctively want to have more cleanliness and clarity in your life.

Make cleaning your makeup and self-care tools part of the mindful beauty process.

Taking better care of ourselves also means taking better care of our everyday tools. Mindfulness reminds us that every aspect of life, no matter how small, is valuable. Being engaged at every step of the self-care process, from the sublime to the mundane, is worthwhile and helps us to bring clarity to our lives.

Brushing Up Exercise

Collect your makeup brushes. One by one, take each brush and examine it with care. Note the condition of the brush and whether it needs to be replaced. Notice if the bristles have become clogged or worn, and whether the brushes meet your self-care standards. Throw away any brushes that are harsh on your skin.

Clean each brush under warm, running water. Make sure the temperature is not too hot for your hands. Allow yourself to fully experience the water falling over your fingers and the brush. Notice the change in texture of the brush as the water cascades through the bristles and it changes from dry to wet. Note how each of your brushes feels to your touch and whether they feel different from one another. See if the water changes color in your hands as you wash the brush. Wash it until the water runs clear. Notice if you can feel other textures or sensations, such as particles or residue in the brush as you wash it. Be aware of how that feels.

Next, fill a bowl with warm, soapy water. Use only a soap or shampoo that is comfortable on your skin. Immerse your brushes one by one in the bowl of water and swirl. Swirl clockwise. Swirl counterclockwise. Swirl large circles. Swirl small circles. Watch the ripples in the water extend from the center, like a stone thrown in a pond. Take more time if you want to. Soak all the brushes in the water for up to thirty seconds.

Remove the brushes from the bowl of water. Take each brush and rinse it under cold, running water. Notice how the different water temperature feels on your hands. Thoroughly rinse out the soap/shampoo. Mold the bristles of the brush back into shape with your fingers, making sure the bristles are all going in the same direction. This will seal the bristles.

Allow the brushes to dry flat, preferably in sunlight.

Alternatively, you can use a professional brush cleaner that comes as a spray. They are available in most drugstores and beauty supply stores. Aromatherapy brush sprays are also available. Brush cleaners refresh, sanitize, and condition both natural and synthetic brushes. To use, spray the cleaner onto a tissue then gently wipe off the excess dirt and debris from the bristles of your brush. Rinse the brushes, then lay them flat to dry.

Contemplate Your Chores

Your cosmetic brushes aren't the only things that can benefit from your mindful care. Choose any self-care enhancing chore, from scrubbing the shower to tidying your cosmetic bag, and choose to do it mindfully. Engage in the task fully. Notice how direct experience of the chore makes it seem like, well, less of a chore. By engaging mindfully in day-to-day tasks you can achieve a sense of spaciousness in your physical and mental surroundings.

Quick Lift: Zip It! Put It in Your Beauty Bag

A way of treating anxiety is by using a worry tree. Writing down your worries or putting them up out of reach in a mental tree, is a useful method. Try this with any appearance-related anxieties. Write down your concerns and put them into a beauty bag or cosmetic case. You can do this literally or in your imagination. Then, zip it! Close the bag. You can deal with it later by taking out and considering one worry at a time and taking action on it at a time when you're calm and relaxed. Your worries will appear very different then.

The Secrets of Mindful Beauty

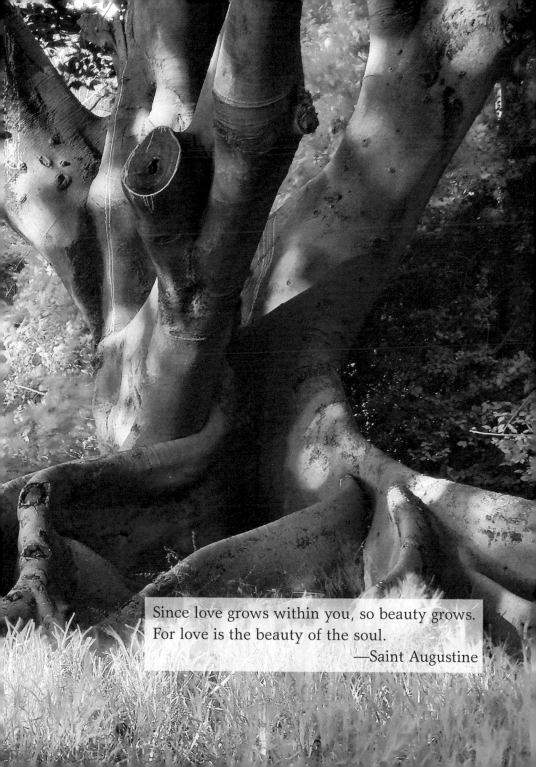

Since love grows within you, so beauty grows. For love is the beauty of the soul.
—Saint Augustine

7 Relax into Beauty

Your total well-being affects your appearance far more than you realize. If you're not balancing your life, it shows. A busy work schedule, lack of exercise, and a poor diet all affect our levels of stress hormones, such as cortisol and adrenaline, which can take a toll on our skin, hair, and nail quality. Poor self-care behaviors can do cumulative collateral damage over time. Just as bad habits can creep up on you, good habits can too. This chapter provides you with holistic methods of relaxation to balance your lifestyle and improve your overall well-being. Relaxation and meditation are cornerstones of mindfulness. Try these relaxation and meditation techniques to bring you into a state of mindful beauty.

Lighten Up: Muscle Relaxation
Muscle relaxation is a great way to reduce stress, helping both the body and the mind relax. We often hold muscle tension in areas of our body without even noticing, such as our stomach, shoulders, jaw, or face. This relaxation exercise works gradually through each muscle group, exaggerating the tension, and then releasing it, allowing for a complete relaxation of the muscular system. With regular practice (even just ten minutes a day) physical strain can be eased, and the mind can be calmed.

- Sit or lie down somewhere quiet and not too hot or cold.
- Start by closing your eyes and paying attention to your breathing. Count through five breaths, noticing the rise and fall of your chest, and seeing if you can expand your breath to the bottom of your abdomen.
- Tighten and release different parts of your body in turn, starting with your toes. Move to your feet, tightening and releasing. Then, move to your legs, abdomen, shoulders, and so on throughout your body. Include your face muscles, jaw, mouth, and eye area. Take time with each muscle group, holding the tension for two to three seconds, and then releasing, feeling the muscles loosen and relax with your exhale. Perhaps you notice some small aches from where you were unknowingly holding tension. Allow this to be part of your experience, feeling that tension and pain soften and subside.
- Now, move your focus back to your feet. Imagine a ray of light moving slowly upwards, through the bottom of your feet, up through your legs and thighs, into your torso, down the lengths of your arms, and up your neck, until the light reaches the top of your head and continues shining upward and outward. Picture yourself aglow and shining with this light.
- Finish the exercise by returning to your breathing, counting your breaths slowly and drawing your breath deeply into your body.
- It's very normal to find your mind wandering during a relaxation exercise like this. If you notice your thoughts drifting back to something that's worrying you, or something you have to do later, acknowledge the thought and gently return your focus to your breathing.

Calm Down: Soothing Meditation

This is a meditation that can be used to soothe the mind and body. This is the aim of meditation: to reach a point at which you are able to still your mind. Many people think they're never going to be able to still all their thoughts, and they're right. Meditation is not about emptying your mind, or getting rid of thoughts. It's about finding a calm center point and simply letting the thoughts come and go, washing over and around you.

- Sit or lie down in a comfortable, quiet place. Ensure your meditation posture is correct: this simply means keeping your spine straight. Try not to slouch or curl your body.
- Close your eyes. To begin, you can use a relaxation exercise, such as releasing muscle tension as outlined previously. Move through the areas of the body where you usually notice tension and release it.
- Now, focus on your breathing, putting your attention on the place in your body where you sense your breath the most: this may be breathing in and out of your mouth or nose, the rise and fall of your chest, or the movement in your diaphragm (refer to the "Finding Your Breath Home Base" exercise in Mindful Beauty Treatment 2, page 42). Some people like to use a mantra to focus. A mantra is a word or phrase, such as "peace" or "let go," that you repeat in your mind in order to achieve the soothing experience you wish to create.
- As your body starts to still, allow your mind to still also. If you notice thoughts enter your mind, try not to follow them. Let them glide by as you continue to breathe slowly in and out. Just keep your attention on the still point within.
- When you maintain the attitude of meditation, eyes closed and letting your thoughts glide by, your breathing will start to slow and you can experience a deep inner calm. This inner calm is having a positive effect on every cell in your body. Feel that calm spread through you.
- Maintain the position for as long as you can, slowly increasing the length of time. Start with ten minutes, increase to twenty minutes, and then up to thirty minutes. Eventually, you may even find an

The Secrets of Mindful Beauty

hour or more slips by. When you've reached the meditative state, you'll see the effect on your face when you've finished. You will look more serene, and your eyes will be brighter.

Practice meditation as often as possible. This might be daily, or maybe it is only once a week. That is okay. Find the level that is right for you and be accepting and patient with yourself. As you continue with mindful beauty, you'll see there are other meditations for you to discover and enjoy. If you do start with once a week, perhaps you can build up to once a day, for a few minutes at a time. You'll soon find you don't want to do without it. Through regular practice, you will be able to bring this calmness into your everyday life. No matter what is going on around you, no matter how much is happening and how stressful it is, you'll be able to find that still point of deep calm within.

Hand Cream Exercise
This is a short mindfulness exercise that can be done almost anywhere, assuming you have some hand cream handy. Keep some near you at home, at work, and in the car. If you are engaged in negative or troubled thoughts, use this to break the negative thinking circuit.

Take the hand cream and apply a small amount in the center of one palm. Start by noticing the color of it, and the contrast with your skin. Notice the temperature, does it feel cool or warm? Slowly begin to smooth the hand cream into your palm. Notice the sensation it creates in both hands. Smooth the hand cream up along each finger and along the backs of your hands, paying close attention to the sensations. Is the scent of the hand cream reaching you? Do your hands feel smoother, more supple? Are they warmer than before?

Try this exercise whenever you want a brief, self-soothing way of engaging with your senses. Use it to break negative thought patterns and as a reminder to be kind to yourself.

Quick Lift: Jaw Tension Release

When we're tense, we often carry it in a particular part of our face or body. For many people, it's their jaw. Clenching your teeth and holding your jaw tight can lead to a tense expression that can eventually "lock" lines and wrinkles into place.

To release the lock:

1. Rest your tongue gently on the roof of your mouth. You will instantly notice a release of tension in your mouth and jaw area. Rest your face in this position as much as possible.

2. If you're feeling very anxious or panicked, press your tongue against the roof of your mouth more firmly. Slowly count to ten, then release. Your breathing will immediately begin to slow down. Repeat three times.

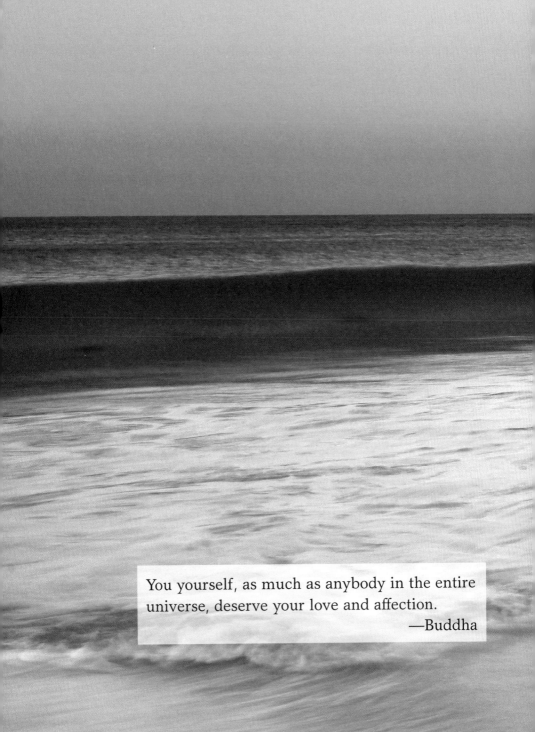

You yourself, as much as anybody in the entire universe, deserve your love and affection.

—Buddha

8

How Do I Look?: Target Ugly Thoughts

Do you find yourself racing to the mirror many times a day to check how you look? Do you find your thoughts always drifting back to the freckles you hate or the frown lines you can see developing? Do you have a feature you especially dislike and think about constantly?

It doesn't have to be like this. Breaking unhelpful thinking habits will help you fight an attack of "the uglies."

Remind Yourself: What's the REAL Problem?

One of the first steps in challenging appearance-related anxious thoughts is recognizing that it is part of anxiety behavior. You're not just obsessively worrying about wrinkles or a blemish because of the wrinkles or the blemish, you're worrying because you worry a lot! Reducing your overall anxiety means the specific form of your worry will stop taking center stage. And the less you worry, the better you'll look.

Whenever you start feeling anxious about how you look, remind yourself: *Worry is the problem, not my wrinkles, my nose, my hair, etc. I can do something about my worry.*

Spend some time identifying what your appearance anxiety thoughts might be and when they usually occur. Focus on the appearance-related thought that most worries you. Prepare your own reminder statement like the one above to replace it. Use it whenever anxiety about a particular issue arises.

See the Whole, Not the Body Part

A tendency to focus on a particular feature or body part, such as your nose or skin, can be very detrimental to your overall well-being. This tendency can lead to exaggeration of a problem, increasing the concern that goes along with it. When you find yourself staring or focusing on one particular feature, remember, nobody else sees just this feature when they look at you; they see your whole self. In fact, most of the time, the feature you are so concerned about may completely escape the notice of others. Instead, try and broaden your thoughts to your whole self—remember to include your wonderful personality! You're not a big nose walking around. You're bigger than a blemish. Don't break yourself into body parts. See and celebrate your whole self.

Break the Ugly Thought Cycle

Negative appearance-related thoughts can be so much a part of our routine that they are almost automatic. They can become a cycle that seems out of control, but with this simple four-step process you can halt the ugly cycle.

- **Recognize** the ugly thought
  Catch yourself in the process of unhelpful thoughts and behaviors. For example, you may feel anxious when you don't look your best. You may spend the whole day thinking, *I look terrible today*, or even alter your behavior, such as avoiding going out or interacting with other people, because of it. You might berate yourself over what you could have done differently, wishing you had gone to bed earlier the night before or hadn't eaten that junk food.

What's hidden beneath the ugly thought? Identify the belief that is permanent and specific to you. Some of these beliefs might be extreme, global, and inflexible. For example, if you think you have to always look your best, ask yourself why? Is it your belief that you must look good every day? Or perhaps you think you should be looking perfect all the time. Now ask yourself if these beliefs are accurate. Do they really reflect the way life is, or have these beliefs become an unhelpful alteration to the way you view life?

- **Dispute** the ugly thought
  Find some evidence to the contrary of your ugly thoughts and beliefs. For example, you may think, *I look terrible today*, and your underlying belief is: *I should always look my best*. Dispute it. Nobody is able to look perfect or great all the time. For every photograph of a celebrity looking good on the red carpet, there is one (or more) online of them looking awful. Think about your friends and other people you know. Is there anyone who looks flawless twenty-four hours a day?

- **Reattribute** the ugly thought
  Excuse me! You're allowed to interrupt, politely but firmly, when an ugly thought approaches. The next step in breaking the ugly thought cycle is called reattribution, which means finding a different explanation that can interrupt your old beliefs. For example, you might tell yourself: It's not possible to look perfect every day. Nobody looks great every day. Everybody has off days.

- **Distract** yourself from the ugly thought
  Switch your focus. Mindfulness is a great way to do this. In this final step, remind yourself that ruminating on ugly thoughts is ineffectual and unhelpful. When you are starting to recognize these thoughts, repeat your reattribution and let the initial thought loosen its grip.

Choose instead to focus on the present, where you are here and now. See below for a quick tip on how to reengage with the present moment.

Recognize. Dispute. Reattribute. Distract. Don't let the uglies beat you!

Quick Lift: Notice Three Things

This is a simple exercise that will help you refocus with the present moment when you find yourself getting caught up in thoughts and worries, especially about your appearance. When you notice yourself doing this, shift your attention to your external world by engaging with it through your senses.

What are three things you can see? Name them in your head. Perhaps pick things of a specific color or theme. Now notice three things you can hear. Let the sounds come to you rather than hunting for them. Listen for a while, then move on to the next one. What are three things you can feel? The floor underneath you? The wind if you are outside? The sensation of your clothing touching your skin? Connect with these sensations. What about smell? Notice any sensations that reach you. Suddenly you will find that you are instantly connecting with the world around you. If your attention wanders back to your thoughts, don't worry, this is normal. Just accept them as part of the experience and shift your attention back to the sensations.

The Secrets of Mindful Beauty

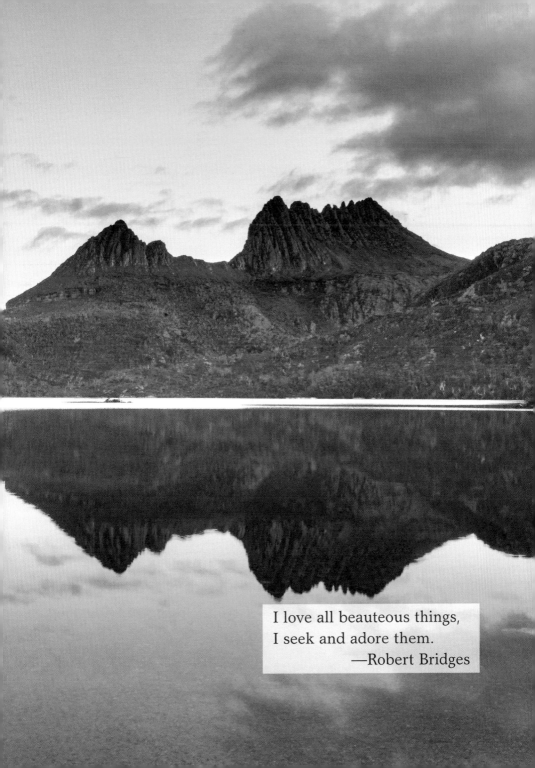

I love all beauteous things,
I seek and adore them.
—Robert Bridges

9 Face to Face with Your Feelings

Our emotions create changes in our bodies, and our bodies create changes in our emotions. Nowhere is this expressed more than in our faces. These fun exercises will help you make the connection and get to know your body sensations. What's happening in your body is often a clue to how you're feeling, so the more familiar you are, the easier you can catch it and choose to respond mindfully. Have you ever noticed you are uptight by realizing your fists are clenched? By uncurling your fingers, you release the tension externally and internally. By getting to know and responding to our facial changes, we can also shift our internal state.

Making Faces Exercise
Do this exercise in front of a mirror.

Happy Face—Make a happy face. Imagine you are meeting someone you love or doing an activity you enjoy. Observe the changes in your face. Your mouth may be upturned into a smile, your cheeks lifted, perhaps your eyes are sparkling. Notice how you feel. Do you feel happy or joyful? Do you sense it in your body?

Sad Face—Make a sad face. Imagine you are saying good-bye to someone you love or watching a sad movie. Observe the changes in your face. Your mouth may be downturned, your cheeks drooping, perhaps your eyes are dulled. Notice how you feel. Do you feel sad or sorrowful? Do you sense it in your body?

Worried Face—Make a worried face. Imagine you are worried about someone you love who is late or you are reading a concerning email or message. Observe the changes in your face. Your mouth is pursed, your cheeks drooping, perhaps your brow is furrowed, or your eyes are squinted. Notice how you feel. Do you feel tense or worried? Do you sense it in your body?

Surprised Face—Make a surprised face. Imagine someone you love has surprised you with a visit, or that you've received some unexpected good news. Observe the changes in your face. Your mouth may be open, your cheeks stretched, perhaps your eyes are wide, lifting the skin of your forehead. Notice how you feel. Do you feel surprised or thrilled? Do you sense it in your body?

Stressed Face—Make a stressed face. Imagine you're running late for an important appointment, have been given an unworkable deadline, or you have too many competing work or family responsibilities. Observe the changes in your face. Your lips may be clamped, your teeth gritted, your jaw clenched. You might be frowning, your eyebrows tightened. Notice how you feel. Do you feel stressed and anxious? Do you sense it in your body?

Calm Face—Make a calm face. Imagine you are in a peaceful place or state of mind, breathing deeply and relaxed. Observe the changes in your face. Your lips may be slightly apart, your mouth relaxed, your tongue resting on the roof of your mouth, your eyes open and alert.

Notice how you feel. Do you feel calm and peaceful? Do you sense it in your body?

Joyful Face—Make a joyful face. Imagine you are enjoying the company of someone you love and they just told you a joke, or you are watching a funny movie. Observe the changes in your face. Your mouth may be upturned into a wide smile, your mouth might be open and your cheeks lifted, or perhaps you are laughing out loud. Notice how you feel. Do you feel happy or joyful? Do you sense it in your body?

Get to know the feelings and sensations different emotions create in your body. Increase your awareness of the mind-body connection. Keep making faces.

Facial Muscle Relaxation
You can make beneficial changes to your internal and external state using the body-mind connection. Work from the outside in with these mini muscle workouts.

Eyes
Do the following without moving your head or the muscles around your eyes.

Roll your eyes upward and count slowly to five. Roll your eyes downward and count slowly to five.

Roll your eyes to the left and count slowly to five. Roll your eyes to the right and count slowly to five.

Roll your eyes down and to the left and count slowly to five. Roll your eyes down and to the right and count slowly to five.

Roll your eyes up and to the left and count slowly to five. Roll your eyes up and to the right and count slowly to five.

Jaw
Make a frightening face. Take your lower teeth and push them up over your top teeth. Hold. Release. Repeat.

Mouth

Turn up the corners of your mouth until you are beaming. A smile has been proven to produce neurological effects on your brain that increase your feeling of pleasure. It's a feedback loop: feel good = smile, smile = feel good. It's so easy it ought to make you smile!

Face Your Feelings Meditation

Make beneficial changes to your internal and external state using the body-mind connection. Work from the inside out with this emotion meditation.

Sit in a comfortable, quiet place. Take up your meditation posture, keeping your spine straight—don't slouch or curl your body. Gently close your eyes and begin to focus on your breathing. We're going to explore your feelings as you meditate.

Focus on your breathing, putting your attention on the place in your body where you sense your breath the most. Rest your attention in that part of your body. Breathe in and out a few times, focusing on your belly. Breathe slowly in and out. As your body starts to still, allow your mind to also still.

In your mind, make a happy face. Don't actually move your facial muscles. Just use your imagination. Imagine you are meeting someone you love or doing an activity you enjoy. Mentally visualize the changes in your face. Imagine your mouth upturned into a smile and your cheeks lifted, perhaps your eyes are sparkling. Notice how you feel. Do you feel happy or joyful? Do you sense it in your body?

In your mind, make a sad face. Don't actually move your facial muscles. Imagine you are saying goodbye to someone you love or watching a sad movie. Mentally visualize the changes in your face. Imagine your mouth downturned, your cheeks drooping, perhaps your eyes are dulled. Notice how you feel. Do you feel sad or sorrowful? Do you sense it in your body?

In your mind, make a worried face. Imagine you are worried about someone you love who is late or you are reading a concerning email or message. Mentally visualize the changes in your face. Imagine your mouth is pursed, your cheeks are drooping, perhaps your brow is furrowed or you're squinting. Notice how you feel. Do you feel tense or worried? Can you sense it in your body?

In your mind, make a surprised face. Don't actually move your facial muscles. Imagine someone you love has surprised you with a visit, or you've received some unexpected good news. Mentally visualize the changes in your face. Imagine your mouth open, your cheeks stretched, perhaps your eyes are open wide, lifting the skin of your forehead. Notice how you feel. Do you feel thrilled? Do you sense it in your body?

In your mind, make a stressed face. Imagine you're running late for an important appointment or have too many competing family responsibilities. Mentally visualize the changes in your face. Imagine your lips clamped shut, your teeth gritted, your jaw clenched. You might be frowning, your eyebrows tightened. Notice how you feel. Do you feel stressed and anxious? Can you sense it in your body?

In your mind, make a calm face. Imagine you are in a peaceful place or state of mind, breathing deeply and relaxed. Mentally visualize the changes in your face. Imagine your lips slightly apart, your mouth relaxed, your tongue resting on the roof of your mouth, your eyes open and alert. Notice how you feel. Do you feel calm and peaceful? Can you sense it in your body?

In your mind, make a joyful face. Imagine you are enjoying the company of someone you love and they have told you a joke or you are watching a funny movie. Visualize the changes in your face. Imagine your mouth upturned into a wide smile, or your mouth open and cheeks lifted. Perhaps you are laughing out loud. Notice how you feel. Do you feel happy or joyful? Do you sense it in your body?

Keeping your eyes closed, without moving the physical muscles of your face, return to the felt-sense in your body that is most familiar and habitual for you, to a face you make a lot. Do you feel happy, sad, worried, surprised, stressed, calm, or joyful?

Which face did you choose?

If you went to an emotion that feels good, there's no judgment in that. Sit with that emotion for a while, practice resting your awareness in that feeling.

If you went to an emotion that doesn't feel good, there's no judgment in that. You can remain with that emotion. Just sit with it, if you can.

When you're ready, you can move back to an emotional state that makes you feel better. You've now increased your awareness and flexibility in your internal emotional range by making faces in your mind. Can you move back to a more positive internal state for a while? You can make the face in your imagination, or you might want to make a face and physically move your facial muscles to help you get there. Make a happy face, a surprised face, a calm face, or a joyful face.

Eventually, by making faces and practicing accessing your emotions in meditation, you will be able to remain sitting with a positive emotion for longer and longer periods. You'll be able to bring that emotion to your mind and body with ease. Your difficult emotions won't disappear—they'll still be there—but you won't need to focus on them. You can acknowledge your difficult emotions, while allowing yourself to remain in a happier state of being. Try to give more attention to the positive emotion than the difficult emotion if you can. If you go back to a more difficult feeling, that's fine. Allow whatever feelings occur to rise up in your mind and body. Accept the full range of your emotions, all the faces you can make. There's no need to avoid them. You can give difficult emotions your attention for as long as you need to, and then return to a more positive feeling when you're ready. Enjoy feeling good, let it move through your body. When you're ready, gently open your eyes.

Do this meditation often, at least once a week. Practice making mental faces. You might discover some additional emotions and faces.

Get to know yourself better and what you're facing inside and out. When you are visualizing, you may find it hard not to move your physical face at first; our mind-body connection is very strong. You may also be amazed to find that even when you just imagine sad or happy faces, you feel those sensations in your body.

Our emotions powerfully impact how we feel, and how we look. We can make choices about which emotions we give our attention to. Positive emotions are always accessible within us. Difficult emotions are always accessible too, but we don't have to stay with them. In meditation and practicing mindfulness, difficult feelings may rise up, and that's perfectly normal. It's by facing them that we create more ease in our minds and bodies. We can then turn our attention to happier emotions that make us look and feel great. About face.

Quick Lift: The Wave of Your Mind

Our thoughts are like waves in the ocean. Going with the current, rather than fighting against the tide, is a useful practice. In mindfulness, this is described as being in flow. If you are surfing or swimming at the beach, the worst thing you can do is struggle against the tide. Let your thoughts be there, but surf them instead. You get to shore by rising above the wave, not fighting it. Go with the flow.

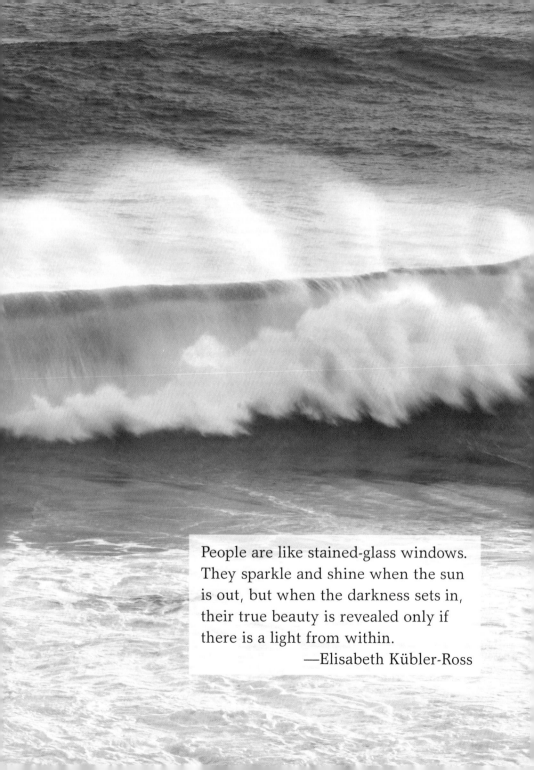

People are like stained-glass windows. They sparkle and shine when the sun is out, but when the darkness sets in, their true beauty is revealed only if there is a light from within.

—Elisabeth Kübler-Ross

10 Imperfect Beauty: Are You a Beauty Perfectionist?

Are you a perfectionist?

What about a *beauty* perfectionist?

While a perfectionist is more generally regarded as someone who has a spotlessly tidy house and not a hair out of place, in psychology the term has a slightly broader meaning. Perfectionists are people who hold high, often extreme standards for themselves. These standards might be applied generally, to lots of areas in their life, or might only be about a specific area, for example work. So, it is possible to be a perfectionist and have a very untidy bedroom!

Appearance and beauty appears to be one of the more common areas where we tend to hold perfectionistic standards. There is so much emphasis placed on perfection in the beauty industry. You don't need to look much further than the names and labels given to products: such as perfect, flawless, and spotless. Accordingly, we tend to expect ourselves to have perfect features, a flawless complexion, spotless skin, and to look our best every day. Similarly, the images we are bombarded with are airbrushed and edited to promote this perfect image. We then expect perfection in ourselves.

Not surprisingly, this can lead to a lot of worry and anxiety when we don't meet this immaculate standard. Another component of perfectionism is experiencing a feeling of failure or distress when these standards are not met. So when our clear complexion is corrupted by a single blemish, this can feel devastating. If we can't get our hair to look just like the example in a magazine, we get frustrated and become angry at ourselves.

Do the above descriptions apply to you? If so, then you might be a beauty perfectionist. Take the quiz below to find out for sure.

Are You a Beauty Perfectionist? Quiz

Answer these questions below to find out if you are beauty perfectionist.

	Very True	Somewhat True	Not True
I expect myself to always look my best.			
If I have a blemish, I feel that I look awful.			
If I have a blemish, I want to stay at home.			
I apply makeup for small outings, such as a quick trip to the supermarket.			
I get upset if I notice I left home with smudged makeup or messy hair.			
I compare myself to images in magazines, even if I know they are airbrushed.			
My physical appearance should be immaculate at all times.			
I hold similar high standards in other areas of my life.			

To calculate your score: Very True = 2 points, Somewhat True = 1 point, Not True = 0 points. Add up your total.

If your score was higher than 9, you might be a beauty perfectionist. Don't worry—it is important to have standards in our lives. However, if these standards become so problematic that they interfere with your life, or drive feelings of inadequacy or failure, you might want to think about loosening some of your tightly held standards.

Battling Beauty Perfectionism—Bring Some Color to Your Thoughts
People with a touch of perfectionism are often prone to *black-and-white thinking*. Black-and-white thinking is the type of extreme thinking that may be behind those high standards we set for our appearance, as we often tell ourselves that if something isn't perfect, then its value is decreased. Examples of black-and-white thinking are: "This blemish makes me look terrible," or, "I always look tired." Words like *always, never, awful*, or *ruined* indicate black-and-white thoughts. We may all be prone to this type of thinking from time to time. Can you think of an example recently for yourself?

There are a couple of ways to tackle these kinds of thoughts. One way is to question the thought and try to find the shades of gray in what we are telling ourselves. Does this one blemish really change your entire appearance? Are other people likely to notice it as much as you do? The answers to both questions are no. Do you always look tired? What about on the weekend when you get plenty of sleep and are well-rested? Spend some time trying to find the spaces between your thought extremes.

Alternatively, if you find that you are often plagued with black-and-white beauty thoughts and finding the gray just isn't cutting it, then try finding the color! Next time you have a beauty-related black-and-white thought (for example, "I have to look my best") try one of the following:

- Imagine the thought popping up on a computer screen as one of those annoying browser attachments and hit the close button.
- Sing the thought to the tune of "Happy Birthday" or one of your favorite Christmas carols (we like "Jingle Bells").

- Say "Thank you, brain!" or "Thanks for the input, inner critic!"
- Imagine your thoughts are encased in a bubble. Watch them rise slowly upward and pop.

These techniques come from work done by researchers and psychologists, including Russ Harris, who authored *The Happiness Trap*. In the book, he provides a number of wonderful ways to play around with distressing thoughts, and see how they can lose their power in the process. You might also like to follow these techniques up with a Quick Lift mindfulness exercise from this book to help you direct your attention back on the here and now, and away from unhelpful perfectionistic thoughts.

A Novel Antidote: Mindful Creativity

Playful. New. Fresh. Bold. Original. Daring. These are words that are inherent in creativity. They aren't part of perfectionism.

Creativity and mindfulness go hand in hand. As you become more mindful, you can also become more creative. A wonderful way to dislodge perfectionism is to allow yourself to be an artist.

We talk about original artworks. Such works haven't followed a template. Likewise, writing a novel is to be engaged in creating something new; the word itself means new. To create a new piece of art, it will be imperfect, because it is different from what has gone before. As we create, we form new ideas of perfection. Every great artist who has ever lived knows that to be true.

Is there an art form that inspires you? Do you long to paint, draw, write, sculpt, sing, or play a musical instrument? No matter which art form you try, let yourself experiment. Try and try again. Allow yourself many mistakes. Create something new from them. The more creative you are, the more artistic and playful you will become about how you look. Every time you allow yourself to be creative and throw yourself into the experience, you are living mindfully and becoming the artist of life you are meant to be.

Quick Lift: Mindful Manicure

One of the biggest contributors to negative thinking is chronic busyness. There just aren't enough hours in the day to get through what you need to do. You're hands-on, 24/7. You're clenching your fists, drumming your fingers, wringing your hands, twisting your rings, biting your nails. Instead of holding tension in your hands, let your fingers have some fun.

- Do some simple hand exercises, especially if you've been working too long on the computer. Close and open your fists and do some finger star jumps: place your palms facing each other. Touch thumb to thumb, index finger to index finger, and so on. Don't let your palms meet. Press your fingers against each other and bend your knuckles, the way you would bend your knees to exercise, and jump! Rotate your wrists a few times to the right, and then to the left. Do some palm presses: place your palms together, press them together tightly, then relax your hands; repeat several times.
- Squeeze a stress ball
- Rub some soothing hand cream into your skin and cuticles
- File your nails
- Enjoy a full or mini manicure

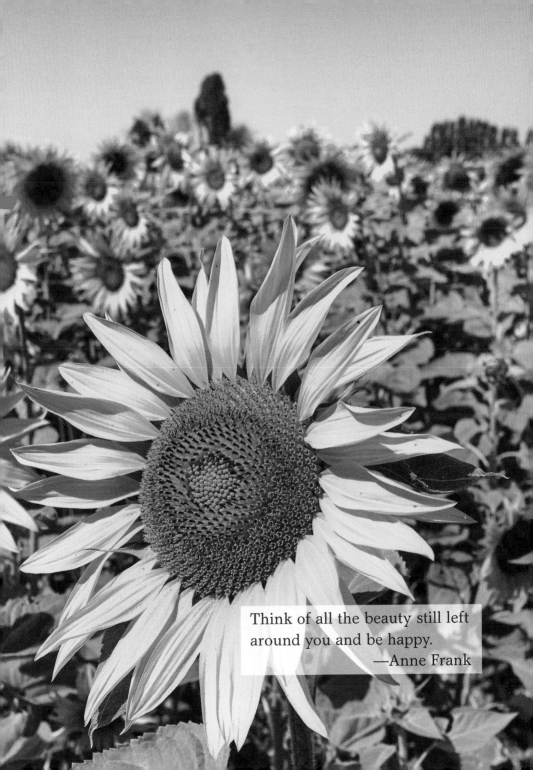

Think of all the beauty still left around you and be happy.
—Anne Frank

11
When It's Not All Pretty: If You Experience Irritation, Continue Use

Stress and depression can make us feel sensitized. It can be compared to having sensitive skin. You know when you've used a cosmetic product that irritates your skin, leaving it sore and stinging, perhaps red and peeling, or even broken or raw. If you're experiencing stress, anxiety, or depression, you're in that tender state of mind.

Mindfulness teaches us self-compassion. Skin care products usually contain a warning: *if irritation develops, discontinue use.* However, mindfulness can bring up some thoughts, emotions, and sensations we can find irritating, and that is NOT a sign to stop. It's a sign to keep going with the process and to learn how to be gentle and kind to yourself, to become more aware and appreciative of who you are. In this chapter, you'll learn some retraining techniques to help.

In Your Sensitive Skin: Learning Self-Kindness from Self-Awareness

As you practice mindful beauty, you will experience increased self-awareness. You'll become more aware of your thoughts, your feelings, and your body sensations. You might be making changes. You might be much more aware of how particular cosmetics feel, whether your skin regime suits you, whether you like your hairstyle anymore. You might even be so much more tuned in to your body that you realize you've got an allergy or sensitive skin and don't want to use certain products anymore. That's the process working. These are some of the beneficial results of your direct experience of discovering you.

You might also be experiencing your feelings more directly—more of them, a bigger range, or unexpected emotions. If you're expecting them all to be good feelings, you may be surprised to discover that your self-awareness brings up some other, less comfortable feelings too. That's normal. Mindfulness doesn't encourage you to ignore any feeling, however you label it. The aim of mindfulness is to give your feeling some space, to notice it. In the very act of noticing it, you are stepping away from it overwhelming you. So notice all of those feelings: anxiety, sadness, resentfulness, anger, dissatisfaction, frustration. Notice when you have them. Notice how they feel in your body. Notice how you label them. Be prepared to give them some attention. Don't stop being mindful because it isn't always pretty. The more comfortable you become with experiencing uncomfortable emotions, the less uncomfortable they become.

If your cosmetic cabinet contains products that irritate or harm you, discard them. The treatment for sensitive skin isn't to keep using painful products. It isn't to rub the skin raw. It isn't to hide away in a darkened room, or shout at your skin to stop being so sensitive and just deal with it. It's the same with negative thoughts and behaviors. Being harsh to yourself, continuing to do things that hurt you, hiding away, or getting angry at yourself—none of that helps. The solution: be gentle, be kind. Being kind to yourself will allow you to recover.

As you grow in self-awareness, treat yourself as tenderly as new skin that's forming. Continue your practice and honor all that it brings up for you. Be as gentle to your psyche and your soul as you are to your epidermis. Gentle, soothing, healing balms: that's what you need most. Calm the inflammation. Soothe those stings. Tend those wounds. Practice self-kindness and let yourself heal.

Attending to Appearance-Related Anxiety

Anxiety is one of the most common uncomfortable feelings women can experience about how they look. A new form of anxiety recently noted by psychologists is what's being called appearance-related anxiety. This form of anxiety, found predominantly among women, is specifically linked to worries about changing appearance, especially due to aging or body image issues. It can be a constant irritation, gnawing away at our self-esteem. Unfortunately, appearance-related anxiety can lead to a vicious cycle, because worrying about your appearance can actually make matters worse. That's why it's so important to address stress at the psychological level.

Cosmetic surgery doesn't necessarily solve the problem. "Fixing" one part of your face, such as your nose, wrinkles, or lips, can often lead to another "fix." It can even lead to a dangerous addiction, with little improvement in self-esteem and happiness. Cosmetic surgery websites often carry warnings that an altered appearance doesn't solve poor self-esteem problems and might not bring about the results sought. That's why boosting your self-esteem through mindfulness is so crucial—no matter what else you do. Use the following mindful beauty meditations to achieve positive self-evaluation and become a believing mirror to yourself.

An Appreciative Glance: Retraining Your Attention

This meditative exercise will help you to train your inner eye to focus more on the positive aspects of yourself and effectively reduce appearance anxiety, unkindness, and irritation. It will also help you to give some room to other challenging emotions.

Sit, stand, or lie down in a comfortable, quiet place. Take up your meditation posture, keeping your spine straight. Don't slouch or curl your body.

Close your eyes and begin to focus on your breathing. Take deep, slow breaths.

Once you are feeling relaxed and comfortable, you can begin.

Keeping your eyes closed, direct your attention to a part of your face or body that you dislike or that feels difficult. What is that part of you? What sensations show up in your body when you direct your attention there? What are your thoughts? What are your feelings? Don't try to change your body sensations, thoughts, or feelings, simply notice what is happening. Keep breathing. Support yourself with your breath.

Now, direct your attention to a part of your face or body that you feel neutral about. What is that part of you? What sensations show up in your body when you direct your attention there? What are your thoughts? What are your feelings? Don't try to change your body sensations, thoughts, or feelings; simply notice what is happening. Keep breathing. Support yourself with your breath.

Next, direct your attention to a part of your face or body that you appreciate, like, or experience positively. What is that part of you? What sensations show up in your body when you direct your attention there? What are your thoughts? What are your feelings? Don't try to change your body sensations, thoughts, or feelings; simply notice what is happening. Keep breathing. Support yourself with your breath.

Practice moving your attention back and forth between these three parts of yourself. Positive, neutral, negative. Negative, neutral, positive. Can you direct your attention where you want it to go? Simply notice the process of movement without judgment. Which area do you pay attention to longer, the negative, neutral, or positive body part? Notice what happens as your thoughts linger in that area.

Now, return your attention to the face or body area you feel positive or neutral about, whichever you find more comfortable. Support yourself with your breath. From this more positive or neutral place, cast a sidelong glance at the part of yourself that you experience as negative. Just look from the corner of your inner eye. What do you notice? Take a quick look, just a glance. See if you can invoke more of a look askance, a question about what you see, rather than a certainty about what you will find. Does the area of concern seem bigger or smaller? More or less important or overwhelming? Notice your feelings and thoughts. Then, if you can, return your attention to the positive or neutral place within you. Keep your attention there. If your attention is drawn away from that positive or neutral place, notice it, and gently return. Repeat this process as often as you like.

Use your breath to funnel your attention—think of it as a laser pointing where you want to go. Make no judgments, just be interested in the process. Experiment with your attention and your inner glance. Direct your inner gaze. Choose to experiment with staying in the place you prefer to be. You are stronger than you know.

When you are ready, open your eyes. Practice this skill whenever you feel appearance anxiety. Simply find a quiet place or moment and close your eyes. Focus your attention on the aspect of yourself you feel neutral about or the part you like. If you can, only give the negative, anxiety-provoking area a quick sidelong glance. The more you practice this skill, the easier it will be. Soon you'll be doing it with your eyes open!

Focusing your attention is a powerful form of mindfulness. There's no right or wrong, just as there are no right or wrong feelings. There is simply an opportunity for you to choose where you want to direct your energy, thoughts, and feelings.

Notice how you feel as you become more adept at choosing where to concentrate. As you continue to practice this skill, you may soon change the percentage of your self-attention. Are your thoughts positive fifty percent of the time? Perhaps you previously focused on your negative aspect more. If you can create more balance, tipping the scales toward focusing on your better or neutral feelings a percentage point or two, you are gaining concentrative mindful power. Just knowing how to do this is powerful.

Give the full benefit of your loving gaze to the parts of yourself you want to look at, that you appreciate, and cast a sidelong glance at the other parts. They won't disappear, but negative feelings and thoughts about those aspects don't have to overwhelm your attention. You can choose where to look. See what happens when you do.

Your First Glance: Seeing with Self-Awareness
Can you catch yourself unaware?

The next time you look in a mirror, identify what you look at first. What do you see at first glance?

Take notice.

Do you look at your face as a whole, your entire body, or do you focus on a particular body part? What are your body sensations as you look in the mirror? What are your thoughts? What are your feelings? Don't try to change your body sensations, thoughts, or feelings. Simply be aware of what you notice when you look in the mirror.

Is it a part that you dislike or experience negatively? What is that part of you? What sensations show up in your body when you direct your attention to that body part? What are your thoughts? What are your feelings? Don't try to change your body sensations, thoughts, or feelings. Simply take note.

The next time you glance in the mirror, see if you can catch yourself in the act of looking. Notice if you can become quicker at catching yourself. See if you can choose what you look at first.

Can you choose to see your whole face rather than a body part?

Can you choose to focus on a part of your face or body you appreciate and like rather than a part you view negatively?

Can you choose to focus on a part of your face or body you consider neutral, rather than a body part you view negatively?

Can you choose to move your attention away from a face or body part that you see negatively? Can you gaze toward a better place or feeling?

You may be surprised at what you see and what you can choose to look at. Your self-awareness is growing. Make no judgments about what you look at first, or if you are slow to change, no scolding or scowling in the mirror. Accept yourself. You have simply formed a habit, and with mindfulness you can shift your focus to what you prefer to see. This choice will reduce the effect of appearance anxiety, because you'll be giving your anxiety less attention, less fuel to guzzle. Your anxiety-provoking aspects won't disappear, but they will have less control over your attention and your gaze. Your inner eye has the power over your eyes. You can choose to appreciate yourself.

In an Instant

Feeling an overwhelming rush of appearance-related anxiety? It's common for this to happen just when we don't want it to, like before a social or professional event.

You can change your mental state in an instant wherever you are and whatever you are doing.

Take three deep breaths.

Now, use your breath to direct your attention away from the anxiety-provoking thought, feeling, or body sensation. Focus it, like a laser, on a face or body part you consider neutral or that you feel good about. Rest your attention there.

Alternatively, direct your attention outward. Focus your gaze and your breath on something around you, a small point of beauty, if you can. (Everything is beautiful in its own way.) Use your laser-like focus to redirect your mind.

If your attention wanders, notice it, and when you can, return your gaze to where you want it to go. Imagine leading yourself gently by the hand. See yourself crouching down next to you and pointing toward something good to look at. Follow that kindly gaze.

With practice you can learn to do this technique in a few breaths. You can do this while doing something else, even in the middle of a conversation. You have the power to focus your breath and your attention right now.

Quick Lift: The Uniqueness of You

This moment is unique. You will never repeat it. You will never wear your hair, apply your makeup, or look the same way ever again. The way your hair falls, the way your eyes light up, the way you smile, all will change in an instant. You are one of a kind. Right now, you are uniquely beautiful. Take a moment of appreciation to glance at your reflection in the mirror or close your eyes and lightly brush your hands over the contours of your face with your fingertips. Notice the uniqueness of you. Cherish yourself in this moment.

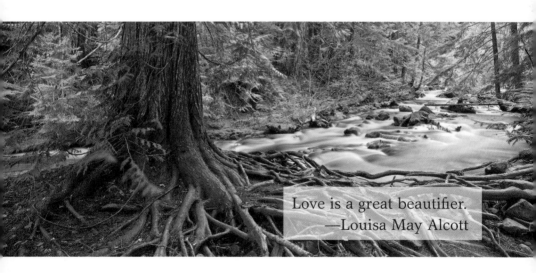

Love is a great beautifier.
—Louisa May Alcott

12 Anti-Aging Stress Management

Suppressed stress boils away beneath the surface of our skin, damaging our health, mind, and bodies. It can make us burst our blood vessels and want to tear our hair out. There's no point suppressing your feelings of stress—that could do more damage—but you can learn how to manage stress with mindfulness.

To disengage from a potentially stressful scene or angry thoughts that won't let go, take some time out for yourself. Set yourself a cooldown time limit before you engage with any provocation. Instead, focus on some soothing self-care and relaxation.

Many women use beauty appointments and spa escapes as a time-out from their busy schedules. They're a great opportunity for mind and body relaxation. Next time you're having a manicure, facial, massage, or spa treatment, use some of your appointment time to be mindful. Pay extra attention to your body sensations. Immerse yourself in the experience, fully attend to it. Appreciate every moment and notice if you enjoy it more. Use your escape to get closer to yourself.

You can also take some time in the privacy and relaxation of your own home with these mindful beauty techniques.

From Time to Time

What do beauty therapists and Buddhist monks have in common?

They both use timers.

One of the elements in being able to relax during a beauty treatment is that the therapist sets the time frame. You don't have to watch the clock. All you need to do is relax.

It's the same with Buddhist meditation. Sessions are often timed—some are long, some are short—and a gong will be struck when the session is over. This allows for a deepening of relaxation and experience.

Occasionally you may wish to use a timer when you are meditating and practicing mindful awareness in your beauty routines. Set a timer for an appropriate time period. You'll notice an enhanced experience, and you will comfortably increase the length of the sessions as time goes on.

Beneath the Mask: Face Mask Meditation

This simple meditation will deepen your experience and self-awareness while using a face mask. Use it with the face mask of your choice. You can carry out this revealing meditation at home or in a salon.

While Applying the Face Mask

As you prepare to apply this mask, prepare to recover the beauty in you.

Cleanse your skin with gentleness. Remove all traces of makeup, leaving your skin damp and clean. Prepare to be fresh-faced and fully open to this experience.

As you apply the mask to your skin in smooth, gentle strokes, notice its consistency, scent, and texture. Apply it evenly and with care, noting any directions for use, such as to avoid the eyes or lips. Pay attention to the mask's purpose, whether it's to soften, smooth, strengthen, nurture, or protect.

While Using the Face Mask

As you use the mask, let it cover your skin. As it sinks into your pores, think of the many masks you wear in your life and the many roles you play.

The mask you wear at work.

The mask you wear at home.

The mask you wear with your family.

The mask you wear in your friendships.

The mask your wear in your relationships.

The mask you wear in the communities to which you belong.

Consider each of these masks in turn. Tune in to your body sensations as you come face to face with each mask. Pay attention to any emotions they evoke. Allow yourself to experience these emotions beneath the safety of the mask now covering your face.

Choose not to judge the masks you wear as good or bad. Each of these masks is part of you.

As this face mask works, sense it on your skin. Feel the mask on the surface of your forehead. Feel the mask on the surface of your cheeks. Feel the mask on the surface of your chin. Feel the mask on the surface of your neck. Feel the mask on any part of you where it has been applied.

Sense the renewal of yourself beneath this mask. Sense the self-care, love, and protection you have applied. Relax into this love and protection, in self-care and silence. Be yourself.

(Leave the face mask on for as long as indicated in the directions.)

While Removing the Face Mask

As you remove the mask, be mindful of the revelation of your face. Notice its contours, its color, and its shape. Notice the work the mask has done in softening, smoothing, or strengthening your skin. Tune in to your emotions about what you have uncovered. Allow yourself to feel nurtured and protected. Accept any other feelings that arise.

As you gently and carefully wash away the traces of the mask from your skin, consider your self-revelations. Wash away any masks you no longer wish to wear in your life, at work, at home, in your family, in your friendships, in your relationships, or in your communities. As you wash the mask away, accept yourself as you are.

Be fresh-faced and open to revealing yourself and the beauty within, beneath the mask.

Windows of the Soul: Extended Eye Mask Meditation
This meditation will deepen your body-sense and emotional awareness while using an eye mask. Use it with the eye mask of your choice. You can carry out this tension-relieving meditation regularly at home or in a salon.

The eyes are called the windows to our souls. The eyes express our emotions. They light up when we smile and weep when we are sad. They are how we see the world. They are important areas of muscle tension or relaxation that have a long-lasting impact on our faces.

Select the eye mask of your choice. It may be a lotion or cream, cooling or comforting and warm. It may simply be a scarf or cloth eye mask to bring your eyes some rest for a short time.

Lie down to apply your eye mask. Assume a relaxed posture, whatever is most comfortable for you.

Close your eyes and take three slow, deep breaths.

Turn your attention to the quality of the mask you have chosen. Observe whether it is soft against your eyes, if it is scratchy, or if there are any other sensations. It may be cool or warm. Observe the area where you sense it most, whether it is most noticeable against the bone around your eye or the socket. Observe the darkness created by the eye mask, whether or not it's still possible to see glimmers of light. Does the mask have a texture? Does it have a scent? Fully engage your senses to experience this eye mask.

Now, turn your attention to your right eye. Fully attend the experience of the mask on your right eye. Tune in to your body sensations. Observe whether you experience these sensations as positive, neutral, or negative. Is your right eye comfortable? Are the muscles relaxed or are you experiencing some discomfort or tension around your right eye? Are you squinting? Allow yourself to fully experience these sensations.

Keeping your attention on your right eye, notice if you experience any particular emotions. It's quite common to experience some unexpected emotions with this level of close self-attention. Observe whether you label these emotions as positive, neutral, or negative. Is your right eye crinkled, calm, or relaxed? Are you experiencing some discomfort, perhaps a sense of sadness, strain, or tearfulness around your right eye? Allow yourself to fully experience these emotions.

When we turn our full attention onto one eye, we can be amazed by what we sense and feel. Now observe where in your right eye you experience sensations and feelings most strongly: is it above the eye, beneath the eye, around the eye? How far do these sensations spread around your eye? Does it stretch up to the side of your head, across the side of your face, or down your cheeks? Allow yourself to experience those feelings and sensations.

Now, turn your attention to your left eye. Fully attend the experience of the mask on your left eye. Tune in to your body sensations. Observe whether you experience these sensations as positive, neutral, or negative. Is your left eye comfortable? Are the muscles relaxed, or are you experiencing some discomfort or tension around your left eye? Are you squinting? Allow yourself to fully experience these sensations.

Keeping your attention on your left eye, observe if you experience any particular emotions. Do you experience these emotions as positive, neutral, or negative? Is your left eye crinkled, calm, or relaxed? Are you experiencing some discomfort, perhaps a sense of sadness, strain, or tearfulness around your left eye? Allow yourself to fully experience these emotions.

Our sensations and feelings can be very different from one eye to the other. Observe now where in your left eye you experience sensations and feelings most strongly; is it above the eye, beneath the eye, around the eye? How far do these sensations spread around your eye? Does it stretch up to the side of your head, across the side of your face, or down your cheeks? Allow yourself to experience those feelings and sensations.

Turn your attention to the spot between your eyebrows. Fully attend to the experience of the mask between your eyes. Tune in to your body sensations. Observe whether you experience these sensations as positive, neutral, or negative. Is the skin between your eyes smooth? Are the muscles relaxed, or are you experiencing some discomfort, tension, or frowning between your eyes? Allow yourself to fully experience these sensations.

Keeping your attention in this spot, notice if you experience any particular emotions. Do you experience these emotions as positive, neutral, or negative? Is the area between your eyes calm and relaxed, or are you experiencing some discomfort or strain there? Allow yourself to fully experience these emotions.

You are now more aware of where your eyes hold strain or tension. By carrying out this process regularly, you'll notice more easily any habitual movements you make around your eyes and be able to address them.

Now let's relieve any tension around your eyes.

Turn your attention to your right eye. Take a deep breath and direct it toward your right eye. Allow the area around your right eye to relax. Consciously let go. Imagine your breath filling the eye socket, like a balloon. Keep breathing: in, out, in, out. With each breath, release the tension around your right eye a little more.

Now, turn your attention to your left eye. Take a deep breath and direct your breath there. Allow the area around your left eye to relax. Consciously let go.

Imagine your breath filling the eye socket, like a balloon. Keep breathing: in, out, in, out. With each breath, the tension around your left eye releases a little more.

Turn your attention between your eyes. Take a deep breath and direct your breath to the area between your eyebrows. Allow the area to relax. Consciously let go. Imagine your breath lightly brushing the skin between your eyes. Keep breathing: in, out, in, out. With each breath, the tension between your eyes releases.

Repeat this process as many times as you'd like. Notice any changes or differences in your eyes. Remember how it feels. You can close your eyes and breathe this way whenever your eyes need relief.

Turn your attention for the last time to your right eye. Without creasing any skin or creating any muscle tension around your eye, fill your right eye with a deep smile. Imagine you are smiling at someone you love without moving a muscle, but communicating that love through your right eye.

Turn your attention for the last time to your left eye. Without creasing any skin or creating any muscle tension around your eye, fill your left eye with a deep smile. Imagine you are smiling at someone you love without moving a muscle, but communicating that love through your left eye.

Turn your attention to both eyes. Without creasing any skin or creating any muscle tension around your eyes, fill both eyes with a deep smile. Imagine you are smiling at someone you love, without moving a muscle, but communicating that love through both eyes.

Let that deep smile fill your whole body with compassion and love.

Breathe that smile.

Sense that smile.

Feel that smile toward you.

Hair-Trigger Temper: Stress Busters

If your anger feels as if it is about to explode from the top of your head, take immediate action.

Stress Head Massage

Massage is a relaxation method that you can do yourself. For on-the-spot relief, try this easy stress buster and soothe away stressors with magic fingers.

Put your hands on either side of your head. Start at your hairline and stretch out your fingers. Place your pinkies near the front of your head, but not onto the skin of your face. Place your thumbs toward the nape of your neck, and the other fingers with an equal distance in between. Press your fingers into your scalp and roll the pads of your fingers in a soothing motion, massaging your scalp. Notice the sensations this creates across your scalp and neck. Slowly move your hands up your scalp, massaging as you go, until you reach the crown of your head. Reverse, slowly bringing your fingers down as you continue to massage. Repeat three times.

(S)tress Time-Out
For instant stress relief, take some time out with your tresses:

- Brush your hair for one hundred strokes, counting slowly.
- Try a new hairstyle. Experiment with curling irons, curlers, and extensions. Play in front of the mirror.
- Stay home and wash your hair. Use your favorite conditioning treatment or oil. Take your time.
- Book an appointment with your hairstylist for a wash, style, or cut.
- Walk out of the problematic situation and walk in to a local hairdresser. Explain that it's a hair emergency. Even if you can't get an appointment, the walk will do you good.

Sensing Beauty
Engaging our senses instantly brings us into the present moment and can relieve our sense of stress, anger, or anxiety. For a speedy stress solution, mindfully indulge one or more of your five senses.

Seeing beauty—Take a few moments to gaze at something beautiful in your line of sight: a flower, a plant, a view, a passing scene. Keep a postcard with a beautiful picture handy, or put a photo that uplifts you onto your phone or computer. Stop and stare for a while.

Smelling beauty—Inhale a beautiful scent. Spray your favorite perfume or room spray around you, light a fragranced candle, or use an oil diffuser. Imagine it as a cloud of protection, an invisible stress-shield. Breathe deeply.

Tasting beauty—Enjoy a burst of flavor. Keep your favorite bubble gum handy. Chew some just for fun until the flavor runs out. A sugar-free lollipop can also give you some stress-free flavor. Fully focus on the taste experience.

Hearing beauty—Create a de-stress compilation of songs on your phone. Select a couple of favorites that will give you a relaxation trigger. When you're under pressure, listen to a relaxing song or piece of music to soothe the stress and drift away to another sound dimension.

Touching beauty—Keep a tactile soother near you: a smooth crystal, a rough rock, or a swatch of fabric (you're never too old for a cuddle rug). Hold onto this soothing object whenever you need to remind yourself to relax, or, for instant stress release, pet an animal.

Quick Lift: Recite the Mindful Beauty Mantra

A mantra is a syllable, word, or phrase originally used in sacred Buddhist and Hindu practices. A mantra can be profoundly transformational, or simply used as a focal point. When you are meditating, you can speak a mantra aloud or say it silently to begin your meditation, or to deepen your concentration. Reciting a mantra can also help if you are stressed or overwhelmed. As many times as necessary, simply repeat the mindful beauty mantra:

Stay Mindful. Stay Beautiful.

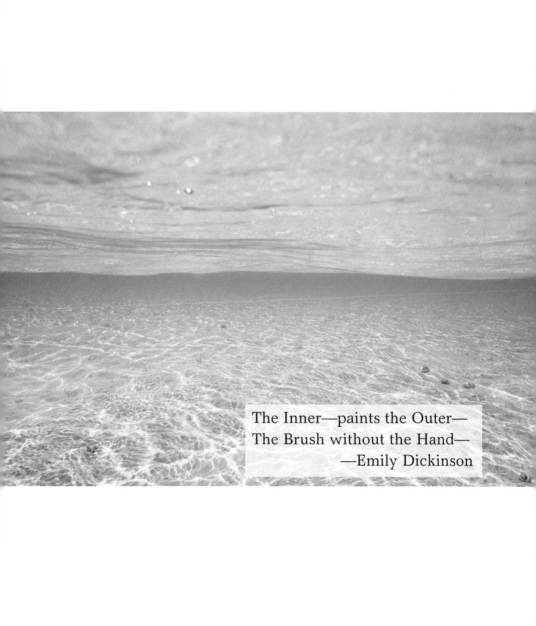

The Inner—paints the Outer—
The Brush without the Hand—
            —Emily Dickinson

13
Silence Your Inner Appearance Critic

Sometimes there can be a bias in regard to the things we tell ourselves. If we tune in to the conversation in our head, we will often find that this voice is typically a critical one. It says things like "You didn't do that well," "You shouldn't have done it that way," "Why did you do that?" This voice (the inner critic) often gets louder when we are feeling fatigued, stressed, or down. The volume of our inner critic gets turned up, and we find that we are berating ourselves throughout the day. Often we are harsher on ourselves than we would be on anyone else, and we might say things to ourselves that we wouldn't dream of saying to others. This isn't a nice way to behave toward ourselves.

Our inner critic can be responsible for a lot. It is the voice that triggers feelings of self-doubt, that keeps us awake at night, that makes us feel guilty for things in the past, and that makes us fearful about things in the future.

Many women also have an inner appearance critic. This unkind variation of the inner critic is the one that speaks to us when we look in the mirror. It points out our flaws. It tells us that we are too fat or too skinny, that we should go to the gym more, that we look awful this morning; it points out the bags under our eyes. The appearance critic is responsible for a lot of abuse.

Awareness of the Inner Critic Exercise

Having some awareness of our inner critic is the first step toward challenging it. Sometimes we can be unaware of how we are talking to ourselves, or if our inner critic is acting up.

During the course of a few days, jot down any statements that you say to yourself. You might notice a pattern. The word "should" might show up a lot. Notice if you are harsher on yourself during certain times of the day in certain situations. Are you harder on yourself in the morning or at the end of the day? When you are out socializing or when you are alone? Take note of this information, as it will become more useful when you are choosing how to tackle your critic.

You might also want to tune in to what your appearance critic says to you. Become mindful of your thoughts. Awareness is the first key. Notice what your critic sounds like and when your critic attacks. Try to catch your critic out!

Balancing the Bias: Meet Your Inner Affirmer

Affirmations can be a way of balancing out some of the negative things we say to ourselves. They are positive statements that we repeat, often while engaging in mindfulness or meditation.

When you find yourself getting caught up in the loud (often insistent) voice of the inner critic, this is a perfect time to try an affirmation. Try choosing a statement that promotes how you want to feel in the situation. For example, if you were doing a quick mindfulness exercise before going into a job interview, you might choose to say, "I am capable and strong." If you are using affirmations to start your daily beauty routine, you might choose to say, "I feel more beautiful with each day that passes." Play around and find an affirmation that fits.

Affirmations work well in combination with breathing meditations. Start with several deep breaths. You'll find more mindful beauty affirmations in Mindful Beauty Treatment 18 (page 154). Try first to develop your own unique, supportive statement to match your unique self. You'll be surprised by what you hear if you let your inner affirmer, instead of your inner critic, have a say.

Affirming Actions Speak Louder Than Critical Words
Your inner appearance critic may never become totally silent. However, you can learn to accept that reality and take affirming action to enhance your life instead. You can turn down the volume and learn to live more comfortably in spite of her constant negative commentary.

Reframe your inner appearance critic as a cosmetic counter assistant who is constantly offering you products or advice you don't want. *No, thank you,* you say politely. Even though you don't want it, she persists. You say *no, thank you,* once again.

When you get caught up in self-critical thoughts, you can't escape that cosmetic counter assistant. She has taken charge! You're sitting in her chair, getting a makeover you don't want. She convinces you that you're lacking in some way, that there's something wrong with you and you need her products to be okay. She is so persuasive that you might even purchase the products she says you need.

You can take some action when you notice the voice in your head is becoming rather insistent and shrill. Your first clue is to recognize that the voice is not your mindful self. Your mindful self is connected to your direct experience, not to self-evaluation. If you're enjoying the experience at the cosmetic counter, that's fine. You might be having a beautiful, mindful moment. But if the inner voice is comparing, contrasting, or evaluating you, that's the sign to step away from that thought. That's right, take a deep breath and back away from that cosmetic counter.

Mindfulness gives you a gap, the moment to choose. When you are mindful, you have a choice whether to listen to that critical voice or to act caringly. When you aren't mindful, many minutes, hours, days, and years of your precious life could be spent listening to the shrill, unhelpful inner appearance critic in your head, when you could be doing something nice for yourself instead.

The Self-Care Solution: Comfort with Loving-Kindness
Choose to take some positive action toward self-care. If your inner appearance critic is constantly judging and bullying you, then it is time to show yourself some loving-kindness with some mindful beauty comforts.

Make mindful beauty your soft place to fall. If someone you knew was being bullied or criticized, you'd comfort them, wouldn't you? When you notice negative self-talk getting out of control, counter it with a few kindly self-care remedies at home or in a salon. The more regular self-caring actions you take in your life, the less power your inner appearance critic has over you.

Mindful Beauty Comforts

Experience:
* a peaceful pedicure
* a mindful manicure
* a breath of fresh air
* a refreshing cleanse
* a fond facial
* a distracting detox
* a hand-holding massage
* a soothing hairstyling
* a gentle exercise
* a sensorial makeup application
* a pat on the shoulder
* a smile in the mirror
* a nice rest

The more you experience mindful pleasure, the less self-evaluation you will engage in. It's one of the benefits of mindfulness. Your inner appearance critic will pipe up occasionally, but she will soon have less to say.

Be comforted.

Quick Lift: Fast Focus on Your Feelings

Find out what you are feeling right now. Stop. Take a few deep breaths. Describe the emotion you are feeling. Name it. Notice whether you label it positive, neutral, or negative. Allow yourself to become fully aware of the emotion. Accept the emotion as it is right now. Take some deep, gentle breaths and sit with this emotion as long as possible for you at this moment. Later in the day, check in on your feelings and notice if the emotion has changed.

The Secrets of Mindful Beauty

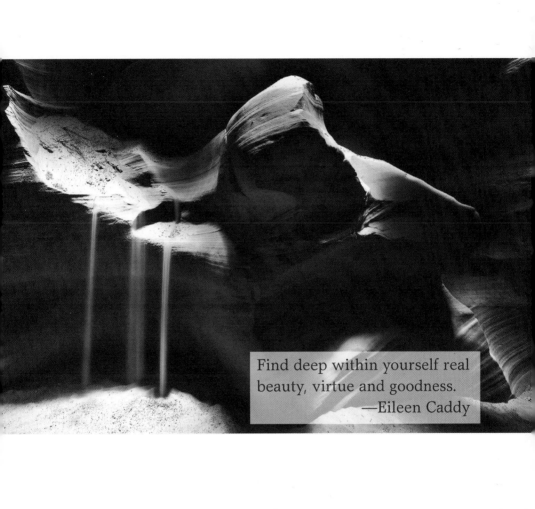

Find deep within yourself real beauty, virtue and goodness.
—Eileen Caddy

14

Beauty Sleep: Better Bedtime Behaviors

The Trouble with Sleep

"How well do you sleep?"

This is a common question asked by many psychologists and doctors, because the state of someone's sleep patterns can tell a lot about their mental state. Stress and anxiety are often the culprits of a bad night's sleep. In particular, worry can keep us lying awake at night, tossing and turning, and unresolved stress and tension can lead to us waking feeling unrefreshed and achy.

Unfortunately, poor sleep can also affect how we look and feel during the day. Sleep is vital for skin repair and increases blood flow to facial areas. So when our sleep is poor, our skin quality is affected, leaving us looking pale and wan. Eye areas can be particularly sensitive to poor sleep, which is why we often have telltale dark circles the next morning. Chronic tension and stress can even lead to nighttime teeth grinding or jaw clenching, which can lead to jaw pain, headaches, and chipped teeth. In addition, when we get too little or poor sleep, the effects show the next day through poor concentration, irritability, brain fog, and emotional sensitivity.

The State of Your Sleep

The state of our sleeping habits can often go unnoticed; for some they can become an ongoing source of stress and concern. Consider the following questions to determine if sleep is an area in your life that might need some extra care and attention.

- Do you lie awake for more than thirty minutes after going to bed?
- Do worry and rumination seem to switch on as soon as you switch off the light?
- Do you have interrupted sleep or disturbing dreams?
- Do you wake up during the night, and then have trouble falling asleep again?
- Does your partner report that you grind your teeth, or do you experience jaw pain during the day?
- Do you wake up with sore shoulders, a headache, or frown lines etched on your face?

If you answered yes to some or all of these questions, you may be in need of some better bedtime behaviors!

Mindful Rituals versus Mindless Routines

One way to address sleep difficulties is by creating a before-bed ritual. This routine can start thirty minutes to an hour before you plan to go to sleep. As we continue a routine, our bodies and minds begin to expect and prepare for bed, so when we turn off the light, we are primed to fall asleep. For even better effects, you can try transforming your bedtime routine into a *mindful ritual*. You will find suggestions for steps and activities in this ritual listed below. A routine can all too easily become mindless habit, whereas a ritual is thoughtful, present, and endowed with meaning. When you were a child, being read a bedtime story was more likely to be a ritual than a routine. Recapture those childhood memories and make bedtime a meaningful part of your day once more.

Try these before-bed mindful rituals to reduce stress and improve your sleep quality.

1. An hour before bed, adjust the lighting in your room or house. Dim overhead lights or switch to lamps. Perhaps light some candles. If you are using a computer screen, consider installing a night-time light filter, as blue light can interfere with the body's internal clock.

2. Take a moment to notice the changes this adjustment in lighting creates. Perhaps colors look softer or less intense. Maybe there is a gentle flicker from a candle flame.

3. Take a bath or shower. While people have preferences about showering in the morning or at night, consider adding a brief shower or a relaxing bath to your before-bed ritual. These can be soothing and relax muscle tension that has built up during the day.

4. Sip a hot drink. Brew some herbal tea or make a warm milk drink to have before bed. Take a moment to mindfully experience it, noticing its scent, the warmth of the cup in your hands, and the delicate taste as you sip it. Feel its warmth move through your body.

5. Take time for makeup removal or a beauty routine. See Mindful Beauty Treatment 1, (page 34) for more suggestions.

6. Spend time making your bedroom inviting and sleep friendly. Close your curtains, perhaps tidy up any clutter that accumulated during the day, keeping your movements gentle and the lighting low. Look around your room and appreciate the calm and peaceful space you have created.

7. Complete a mindful meditation exercise. Try one from an earlier treatment, such as a body scan. This can relax you physically, ease tension, and calm your mind.

   Still noticing the daytime worries? Try a journaling exercise. Journaling can be a great way to empty your head of the thoughts and concerns that have plagued you during the day. Keep a notebook and pen near your bed for this ritual. It can even be used if you find your worries wake you in the middle of the night.

Prayers Before Bedtime: Essential Mantras

With their sacred and healthful properties, essential oils are a marvelous aid to mindfulness and can be a wonderful addition to mindful bedtime rituals, as well as at other times of the day. The sense of smell is often an underutilized means of accessing the present moment, and can be a wonderful, relaxing way to incorporate a gentle mindfulness activity into your nighttime ritual, as well as cue your body for sleep.

Essential oils have long been considered sacred, mystical, and beauty enhancing. Their use goes back more than two thousand years. The ancient Egyptians, Chinese, Greeks, and Romans all used oils. Healthful, healing, and holy, oils have anointed bodies and cleared minds for centuries, and been part of religious practice. Today they're used in aromatherapy and massage, and at complementary health clinics as well as beauty salons. Aromatherapists refer to essential oils as the heart of a plant.

Mantras are another wonderful aid to mindfulness that aims to bring us to the heart of our experience and to our essential selves. A sacred utterance, a mantra is powerfully concentrated. It captures the essence of thought. As with essential oils, in a mantra, less is more.

These mindful beauty essential oil mantras provide a one-word focus point for use with essential oils. They have been selected based on ancient and traditional meanings and uses of the plant. Select an oil and a mantra that fits the state of body and mind you would like to create before sleep; for example, feeling calm, relaxed, or at peace.

As you use the essential oil of your choice, infuse your experience. Breathe in deeply, inhaling the scent of the oil on the inhale. As you exhale, say the one-word mantra. Repeat as needed. Breathe in the essence of beauty.

Mindful Beauty Essential Oil Mantras

Bergamot—Abundance

Eucalyptus—Health

Frankincense—Prosperity

Ginger—Revive

Jasmine—Sweetness

Lavender—Relax

Lemon—Purify

Lemongrass—Cleanse

Marjoram—Comfort

Myrrh—Bless

Orange—Happiness

Patchouli—Connect

Rose—Love

Rosemary—Remember

Sage—Wisdom

Sandalwood—Heart

Thyme—Grace

Ylang-ylang—Peace

Below you will find some additional ways to incorporate the use of essential oils into mindful exercises.

Inhalations

Inhalations are a simple way to bring the vapor of fragrant oil into your life. Oil burners, diffusers, and candles scented with essential oils are easy to use. They can be lit in your bedroom prior to sleep to create a fragrant, welcoming atmosphere.

Steam is another method long utilized in beauty salons. Add a few drops of essential oil into a bowl containing four ounces of hot water. The water must be hot enough to raise steam, but not too hot for your skin. Cover your head and the bowl with a towel and breathe deeply. Repeat the appropriate mindful beauty essential oil mantra. Steam clean your face and mind.

Hand Bath

This soothing treatment can be carried out before a manicure or on its own. Repeat the appropriate mindful beauty essential oil mantra as required. Fill a small basin with warm water and add a few drops of your chosen essential oil. Let your hands rest in the water for a few minutes—steep and swirl. If the water cools, add more warm water.

This simple remedy can be used anytime to soothe and cleanse over-worked fingers. If desired, follow up by gently massaging hand cream into your hands.

Foot Bath

This relaxing treatment can be carried out before a pedicure or on its own. Repeat the appropriate mindful beauty essential oil mantra as required.

Revive those aching feet with oil and water. In a basin or bathtub, add your chosen essential oil to warm water and let your feet soak. Once you're done soaking, take care and dry them well. Add a drop of essential oil to your favorite massage oil and massage your feet. Stay focused as you massage, paying attention to the muscles, joints, and bones that support you every day.

Body Bath

If you love baths, invoke mindful moments by adding essential oils to your bathwater. Bath oil softens and soothes the skin and is an excellent beauty aid. If you prefer showers, add a drop of essential oil to a body oil. While your skin is still wet from the shower, rub on the body oil. It will be absorbed quickly without any residue. Finish your bath or shower with a deep breath and a mindful beauty essential oil mantra.

WARNING: *Always dilute essential oils. Never use undiluted essential oils directly on the skin or in direct sunlight. Avoid use if pregnant and take care with sensitive skin. Do not use on children.*

Quick Lift: Pay Attention

Remember when you were a small child and you wanted your parents to notice you and give you some attention? You can do that today for yourself. If you're overwhelmed, tired, frustrated, or you just don't know how you feel (like a small child gets sometimes) stop and say to yourself, "You have my full attention." Listen carefully to your reply. It might surprise you.

The Secrets of Mindful Beauty

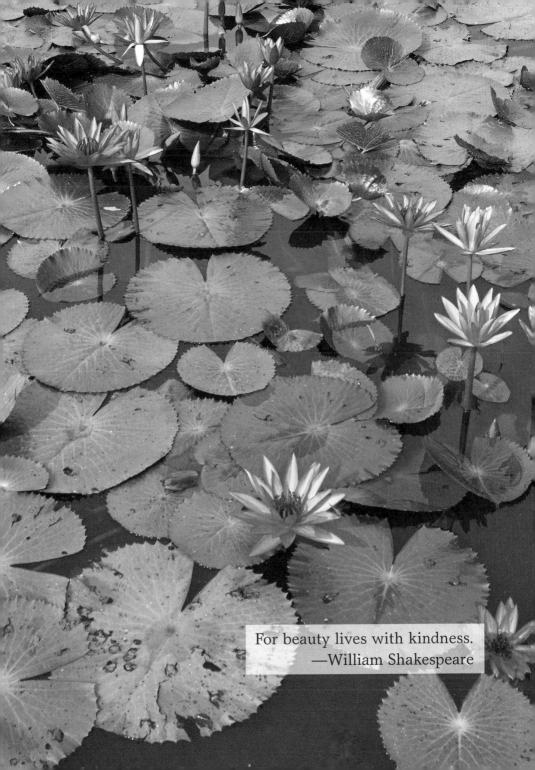

For beauty lives with kindness.
—William Shakespeare

15 See Fifty Shades of Pink: Add a Rosy Glow to Your Life

When we're pessimistic, we see life in fifty shades of gray or become prone to negative thinking. When we're optimistic, we see life in shades of pink. Utilizing the mindfulness concepts of nonjudgment and self-kindness, discover how you can change how you see the world and yourself in a more positive light.

Feel Attractive: Believe in the power of optimism.

Ever noticed how happy, smiley people seem to have happy, smiley lives? It's all right for them, you might snarl, everything's going their way. They have all the luck.

There's a good reason. Optimists aren't happy because they're lucky. Optimists are lucky because they're happy.

This isn't New Age hype or a secret known only to a few. It's psychological fact.

Seeing the good in things actually works, whatever its pessimistic detractors may say. Optimists believe they can overcome adversity, and the important thing is, they act as if they do. They behave their way to success.

Psychological research reveals that optimists have a number of advantages in life.

- Optimists have better overall health.
- Optimists take more chances.
- Optimists complete more tasks.
- Optimists see more opportunities.
- Optimists have more friends.
- Optimists are less prone to depression and other mental illnesses.
- Optimists are less prone to substance abuse.
- Optimists have better relationships.
- Optimists achieve more success.

These advantages are attractive. They're available through action. There's more to it than wishful thinking; there's a big BECAUSE. Here's how it works:

- Optimists have better overall health BECAUSE they attend to their health and well-being. They address any problems early, believing they will be cured, giving a higher chance of a good outcome.
- Optimists take more chances BECAUSE it increases their odds of success. The better the odds, the more likely the positive result.
- Optimists complete more tasks BECAUSE they know that if you don't finish, you can't win the race. Because they finish, they have more wins.
- Optimists see more opportunities BECAUSE they're looking for them. They expect to see good things, so they go out and find them.
- Optimists have more friends BECAUSE they assume they will like others and that they will be liked. They brush off failures more easily.
- Optimists are less prone to depression and other mental illness BE-CAUSE activity, exercise, self-care, and friendship are all part of an optimist's life, which all help keep depression at bay.

- Optimists are less prone to substance abuse BECAUSE they choose to practice self-care and stay positive. They believe they can do without addictive substances.
- Optimists have better relationships BECAUSE happy, enthusiastic people are fun to be around!

These positive benefits are available to you whenever you choose positive life actions instead of negative ones.

In the Pink Exercise

Let the power of positive attraction work for you. No one can expect to feel upbeat and optimistic all the time. It isn't realistic to suggest that everything is rosy, but you can choose to put things in a prettier light.

Whenever you are dealing with a challenging event, person, or circumstance, instead of asking yourself how bad it is, ask yourself how good it is. What shade of pink? Is it blush, magenta, crimson, cherry, coral, cerise, fuchsia, puce, rose, berry, carnation, carmine, champagne pink, pale pink, salmon pink, hot pink, Barbie doll pink, baby pink, shocking pink?

Customize your own personal pink chart so you can adjust how you color the situation. Decide how black you're going to paint it. Stripe it with pink, polka dot it, border it or edge it, make it bloom with flowers, turn it into a sunrise. However pink you choose to make it, change how you look at it.

You're in control of the shades of your life.

Purchase new or select from your cosmetics the pinkest lipstick or lip balm that makes you smile most. Apply it mindfully. Wear your favorite pink shade for a moment or a day whenever you need to see life in a more positive tint.

Put on those rose-colored lips! Get lucky!

Achieve Mastery: Get the Glow of Success

Another powerful way to achieve more positive self-esteem in your life is to take steps toward achievement. It doesn't work the other way around. First the action, then the grace.

Your beauty esteem is connected to your overall self-esteem. At the root of poor self-esteem is the idea of being a failure. This idea is probably added to by a lot of negative self-talk and not-so-constructive self-criticism. You may also accept and internalize criticism from other people, the kind of criticism that people with high self-esteem would let slide by.

There's a way you can actively dispute the idea that you're a failure. It's by achieving mastery. By learning a new skill or improving on one, and achieving a level of success, you build up a powerful bank of positive self-esteem you can withdraw from whenever you need it.

People with low self-esteem often give up easily; they think they can't achieve anything and that trying isn't worthwhile. Perfectionism also prevents us from trying; we think we have to get it right the first time. If you want to get the glow of satisfaction and success, it's time to make a change.

There are three Ps to achieving mastery: practice, patience, and persistence. With these, you cannot fail to gain a level of success. What's more, by practicing mindful beauty, you've already given yourself a better chance of achievement. Mindfulness and meditation increase concentration and can make learning easier.

Master a Makeup Art

A mindful beauty way to mastery is to learn some new beauty skills.

Set aside some time to conquer a beauty trick or technique that you want to improve or that's new to you. Study a book or magazine, watch a YouTube tutorial, visit a cosmetic counter and ask for help, or go to a class. Choose one skill and then add more to your palette. Allow yourself to become absorbed in the task.

Learn, refresh, or polish how to:

- blend foundation for shade and smoothness
- select a blush for your skin tone
- brush and highlight with blush
- sculpt and contour your cheekbones
- define and tweeze eyebrows
- shade and thicken eyebrows
- line, smoke, and smudge with eyeliners
- pencil eyelashes, lids, and brows
- draw with liquids and gel eyeliners
- lengthen or curl eyelashes
- attach fake eyelashes
- create eye effects with shadow
- gild with gold, silver, bronze, and copper powders
- dust and set with face powders
- select a lipstick shade for your skin tone
- draw with a lip pencil
- use a lip brush
- give yourself a manicure
- give yourself a pedicure

Achieving makeup mastery will lead to more creativity and success. Once you've learned or updated some makeup skills, your self-esteem and beauty esteem will have a well-earned boost.

In her book *On Becoming an Artist*, Ellen Langer notes that putting on makeup is a highly creative act. Mindful creativity is a perfectionism circuit breaker, so get creative about your self-care and makeup. How creative can you make it? The more playful you are the less likely you are to require it to be perfect. You'll be having too much fun!

Focus on the process, not the outcome. That's the difference between mindfulness and mindlessness. Remember, you don't have to become the best or do it perfectly. An old master wasn't an artist who followed the rules, but one who transcended them. Just keep on trying until you're satisfied with your level of prowess, and then add your own unique touches. You're going to make mistakes. You're going to want to give up sometimes; it's all part of the process. With practice, patience, and persistence, you'll begin to improve, and you'll begin to feel better about yourself and boost your self-esteem. You're not a failure after all! Achieving mastery in any skill, large or small, means if you start to criticize yourself again, or if someone else criticizes you, you've got positive proof to counteract it. The sheen of success is unmistakable.

Optimize: Open Your Heart

Have you ever seen how your face looks in repose? If the corners of your mouth are droopy or pursed, then it's time to turn that frown upside down. Simply lifting the corners of your mouth will not only help you avoid permanent downward lines, but also give you an instant mood boost.

A form of meditation growing in popularity is open heart meditation. It is a gentle and joyful meditation that increases optimism.

Close your eyes. Place two fingers on your spiritual heart.
(Your spiritual heart is in the center of your chest, just below where your collarbones meet.) Now, touching your spiritual heart, breathe gently in and out . . . and smile.

This simple meditation is both gladdening and calming. It connects you to the emotions you might experience when you are in nature or when you greet someone you love. In open heart meditation, some practitioners use the phrase "smile to your heart" while they meditate to direct their loving attention. It truly is heart-warming. Other practitioners use the phrase "smile, relax, surrender."

Try this simple meditation for a minute or two (or more). Open your heart and bring a smile to your face. You'll be glad you did.

The Mindful Beauty Treatments   137

Quick Lift: The Law of Attraction

Like attracts like. That's the law of attraction. It's a popular idea that we attract whatever comes our way. Being attractive doesn't mean having a particular look or beauty style. It doesn't mean being a specific size, shape, or age. Being attractive means believing you can invite the attention and admiration you desire by first giving it to yourself, just as you are. Try the law of attraction the mindful beauty way. Regularly repeat to yourself the following phrase, "I'm very attractive," and witness as the world begins to agree with you. There's nothing more attractive than self-acceptance.

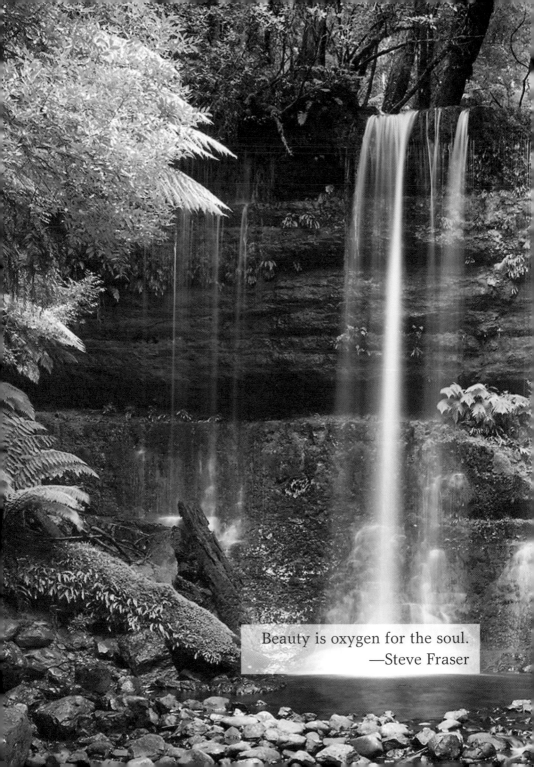

Beauty is oxygen for the soul.
—Steve Fraser

16 Embody the Seasons

Appreciating the seasons brings more awareness into your life. It's also a great beauty boost for your body, inside and out. Noticing the changing seasons of the year allows us to accept and welcome the changing seasons of beauty reflected over the years in our faces and bodies.

Bringing the Seasons into Your Body

To fully embody the seasons, there's no better way than through what we eat. Nutritionists encourage us to naturally bring more vitamins and minerals into our diets by including a rainbow of color. One of the easiest methods to do this is to eat more fruit. Even more mindful is to eat fruit according to the seasons.

Each season offers its own ripe shades and tastes:

Spring: rhubarb, herb greens (mint, parsley, dandelion), pineapple, apricots, oranges (Valencia)

Summer: strawberries, cherries, raspberries, gooseberries, blueberries, peaches, melons (cantaloupe, watermelon), mangoes, apples, blackberries, grapefruit

Fall: pears (late summer/early fall), grapes, plums, quinces, cape gooseberries, crab apples, huckleberries, kumquats, cranberries

Winter: pomegranates, clementines, dates, grapefruit, kiwifruit, oranges (navel), passionfruit, persimmons, red currants, satsuma mandarins, tangerines, lemons

A simple mindfulness exercise is to fully appreciate the gift of each fruit. The Buddhist tradition, from which mindfulness comes, reminds us that we have a responsibility to reflect in ourselves the nature of what we eat. For example, before you eat a rich, golden apricot, acknowledge its beautiful gift to you. Examine its color. Feel its texture, soft or firm. Inhale its scent. Notice its temperature. Is it cold from a refrigerator or warmed by the sun? Have you let it ripen? Taste it. As you eat it, enjoy every juicy bite. When you've finished eating the fruit, give thanks. Honor the fruit you have eaten, the bounty of the earth. Become as rich, ripe, and golden as an apricot. Each season of life brings its own rewards.

Bringing the Seasons into Your Beauty Routine
Bring the changing seasons into your beauty routine through your senses. Each season, select a face, body care, or makeup item that reflects a sense of the season, such as a fresh herbal face mask in spring, a berry-flavored lip balm in summer, a plum shade of lipstick in fall, or a tangerine-scented hand or body lotion in winter. Enjoy selecting it as the weather turns. Stay connected to the fruitful beauty of each season reflected in you.

Self-Love in Season
Mindfulness and creativity have a fruitful relationship. Poets such as Shakespeare often contemplated nature. They were naturally mindful.

Creativity is encouraged by mindfulness, and, in reverse, creativity encourages us to be in a blissfully mindful state.

Many poets wrote about the seasons and used them as a metaphor for love. "Love is not love / Which alters when it alterations finds," wrote Shakespeare. Love is a paradox: it must be constant and true enough to cope with growth and change.

Mindfulness encourages kindness and self-love. Read through the different seasons of life on page 143. They don't last for a set amount of time. They each have different strengths and challenges, but you can choose to be creative. Make whatever stage of life you are in right now your loving season.

Loving Life's Seasons

Spring: We speak of both the first flush of love and the first flush of youth. Life in the springtime is young, new, green. It is exciting, unknown. It is also untried and untested: "Rough winds can shake the darling buds of May," Shakespeare reminds us. Self-love at this stage of life brings newness and freshness, making new discoveries about who you are.

The scent of spring—Give yourself a special gift. Celebrate if you are in this stage of life with a green, leafy scent.

Summer: "Shall I compare thee to a summer's day?" starts Shakespeare's famous sonnet. Summer is life in full bloom. It is passionate, generous, and red hot. Self-love at this stage of life is letting yourself blossom into who you fully are.

The scent of summer—Give yourself a special gift. Celebrate if you are in this stage of life with a lush, floral scent.

Fall: The leaves start to fall away; the person underneath is revealed. "Three beauteous springs to yellow autumn turn'd," as Shakespeare phrased it. This season we begin to see deeper into ourselves, to what is unchanging beneath. Self-love at this stage of life celebrates the fruits we have harvested, and all that is in store for us.

The scent of fall—Give yourself a special gift. Celebrate if you are in this stage of life with an earthy or fruity scent.

Winter: The trees are bare, and we too are bare. There are few leafy illusions left about who we are. In Shakespeare's words again, "Barren winter, with his wrathful nipping cold." The wind may blow cold, storms may come, but we don't need to freeze. For those who celebrate winter, there is warmth by the fire and the wisdom that comes with self-knowledge.

The scent of winter—Give yourself a special gift. Celebrate if you are in this stage of life with a spicy, woody scent.

Quick Lift: Scented

Scent is a stimulating and pleasant way to awaken your senses and bring instant mindfulness. It's all too easy to become accustomed and not notice the scents around us. Our sense of smell diminishes with familiarity. As you go about your beauty and self-care routines, inhale. Remind yourself of the scent of your soap, your shampoo, your body lotion, your hand cream, your lip glosses and balms, and any other scented product. If your products are unscented, smell them as well. They will still have a scent. One by one, lift each product to your nose. Is it spicy, woody, flowery, fruity, or botanical? What does it remind you of? Breathe in deeply. Appreciate the scent of your life.

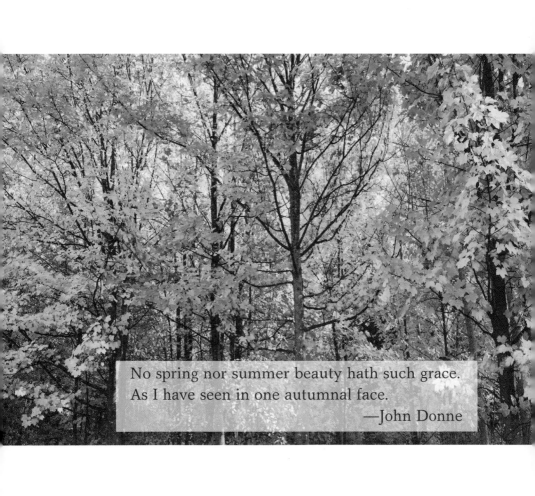

No spring nor summer beauty hath such grace.
As I have seen in one autumnal face.

—John Donne

17 Exercise Your Power: Moves for Body and Mind

Exercise not only improves how you look by increasing your overall suppleness and muscle tone; it's also a powerful bad mood buster. In some cases, exercise has been claimed to be as effective in treating mild to moderate depression as an antidepressant. The positive effects of exercise are also being researched for their use in treating anxiety and other psychological issues. Overall, exercise is a good thing for feeling and looking good.

To maintain an effective self-care exercise routine, choose a sport or activity wisely. Support, don't punish, yourself. Grimacing at the gym, crying with exhaustion at the end of a workout (or before you start), giving up and then beating yourself up about it, or feeling disappointed in your performance won't ultimately help.

Exercise the mindful beauty way. Select an exercise routine for both a physical *and* a mental health boost. Check out whether it helps you to stay in the moment. Let it engage you fully, body and mind.

Exercise for energy: aerobics, dance, cycling, skiing, horseback riding, and running provide a high-impact workout plus a mood and energy high.

Exercise for strength: pilates, ballet, weight lifting, climbing, rowing, and circuit training add to your muscle tone, suppleness, and your sense of power in the world.

Exercise for relaxation: walking, yoga, tai chi, swimming, and golf improve your physical well-being and reduce stress.

Exercise for fun: netball, volleyball, hockey, basketball, and tennis are enjoyable team sports and social activities that enhance your social connectedness and improve mental health too.

Choose an exercise affirmation to give you an extra mindful beauty boost:

- I exercise my body and my mind.
- I am strong and beautiful in mind and body.
- I take good care of my body and my mind.
- My mind and body are flexible and free.
- I grow stronger and wiser every day.
- Strong is beautiful.
- Beauty is powerful.
- I engage fully in life.
- I am supple in mind and body.
- I look good and feel good.
- My body is the temple of my mind.
- I possess mind and body power.
- I am powering up my body and my mind.
- Toning my muscles tones my mind.
- Fit body, fit mind.

Enjoy exercising, but don't overdo it. Stressing your body can increase your cortisol levels with negative cosmetic effects. Push yourself to your limits, but don't go past them. Be mindful. Love your body and mind.

Power Postures

Evidence from psychological literature suggests that standing in certain postures can reduce stress hormones and promote greater feelings of confidence.

One particular study looked at the effect of standing in an open, expansive posture (arms and shoulders wide and open, legs uncrossed, head held high) for a period of one minute, in comparison to closed, low-power postures (arms and legs crossed, shoulders hunched, head down). The study concluded that engaging in such postures may improve people's ability to handle stressful situations, increase confidence, and reduce stress.

Exercise: Paying Attention to Your Posture

Pick several points during the day to mindfully tune in to your posture. You might like to pick different settings, such as at work, during a meeting, talking with a friend. You might be standing or sitting. Notice what you are doing with your limbs. Are your arms or legs crossed? What about your shoulders, are they rounded or hunched? What about your neck? Are you staring at the ground or looking straight ahead? Perhaps you could try shifting your posture slightly, maybe squaring your shoulders or uncrossing your arms.

Jon Kabat-Zinn also describes the meditative stance as a power posture. Whether standing, sitting, or lying down, bringing your mind to attention has energy and purpose.

Embody your power.

Mind-Body Exercises

Give your mind-body a workout with these fast and simple mindful beauty exercises.

Speed Body Scan

Find out what your body is doing right now with a fast body scan. At any time of day you can increase your body awareness and avoid getting into poor beauty habits. Is your forehead tight? Are your eyes squeezed or squinted? Is your jaw clenched? Is your mouth pursed or pressed together? Is your neck drooping? Is there any strain or tension across your back or shoulders? Is your stomach churning? Are your hands clenched? Gently direct your breathing to the area of muscle tension in your body. Take a few deep breaths. Relax. Let go.

In the Palm of Your Hand

When your eyes are tired, tune in to your body's energy by using the palming technique. Briskly rub the palms of your hands together for thirty seconds. You may feel some tingling in your hands. Cup your hands and place them over your eyes. Breathe in and out slowly for one minute. Remove your hands. Blink.

Ear Massage

An unusual mind-body beauty technique is an ear massage. It only takes a minute. Place your thumb behind the top of your ear and your forefinger in front. Working your way down the ear, gently massage the skin between your thumb and forefinger, ending at your earlobe, massaging as you go. According to beauty therapists, your face will glow. What's more, holding the earlobe for a few seconds is a well-known confidence trick. It can help you focus your mind before speaking in public, at a presentation, meeting, or an important event. Celebrities have been known to use it during media interviews. To help alleviate nervousness, make gentle strokes upward on your right earlobe. Reverse the direction and make gentle strokes downward on your left earlobe. Try it and see. You can always pretend you're adjusting your earrings.

Chin-Ups

There's an easier way to do chin-ups than at the gym. Tap twenty times with the flattened back of your hand beneath your chin. This can provoke skin stimulation and encourage you to hold your head high. Chin up.

Quick Lift: Beautiful Music

We all love songs with the word "love" in them, but the word "beauty" comes a close second. There are thousands of songs with the word "beauty" or "beautiful" in the lyrics. Allow a beauty song to come into your mind. You may recall more than one. Sing or hum one to yourself. If you can't think of a song, search online for one you like containing the word beautiful. Download the song and make it your mindful beauty theme song to remind you how beautiful you are.

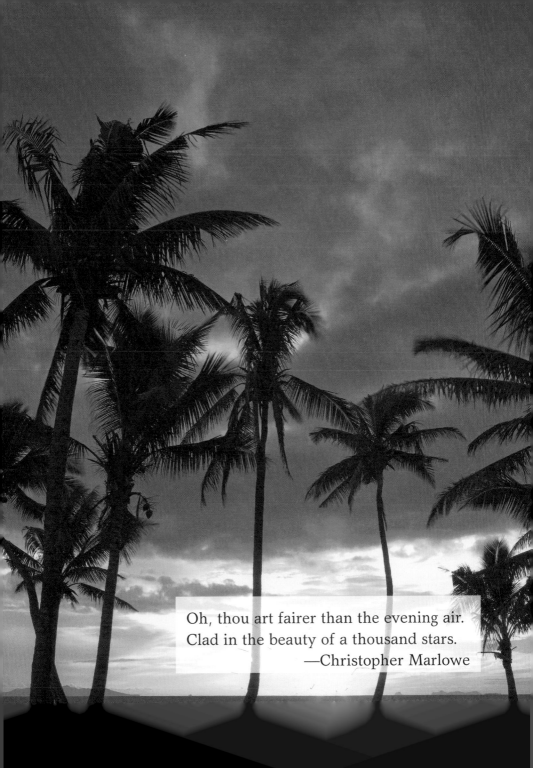

Oh, thou art fairer than the evening air.
Clad in the beauty of a thousand stars.
—Christopher Marlowe

18 Cast a Glamour: Mindful Beauty Affirmations

Glamour Casting: A Spell of Confidence

Glamour is a magical way of seeing. It refers to looking a certain way that creates an impression that is better than the reality. It can include a look of luxury or elegance, or a confidence in style or expression. Glamour incorporates clothing, accessories, makeup . . . and a little bit of imagination.

Glamour also refers to magical beauty or alluring charm. The word has become associated with a magical spell cast on the viewer by the spell-caster to create a more attractive appearance. The word glamour came into use in Scotland, connected with the power of second sight. It was first recorded by poets in the nineteenth century to capture this aspect of beauty and allure.

A "glamour gift" is the skill of enchantment and charm. You can cast this gift into your own hands.

How to cast a glamour:

* **Redirect your gaze.** Use the techniques above to refocus your attention on the face and body parts you appreciate. Concentrate your efforts. Accentuate the positive.

- **See the whole.** A glamour takes in the full face and body. Be whole-minded and full-bodied.
- **Flaunt it.** Whatever you like best about yourself, draw the eye toward it. Let your most positive attribute be the star!
- **Be confident.** Shift your shape. Take up a power posture that is strong enough to contain your glamour. Be sure of your ability to pull it off.
- **Choose a glamorous patroness.** Flick through magazines, watch movies (especially old black-and-whites from the Golden Age of Hollywood), and learn tricks of the trade from the stars. They learned it too, so share their lessons.
- **Invoke the elements.** Do you want to look cool? Invoke water. Choose clothing, accessories, and makeup that conjure the liquid, aquatic element. Do you want to look strong? Invoke stone. Choose clothing, accessories, and makeup that conjure the element of rock and earth. Do you want to look hot? Invoke fire. Choose clothing, accessories, and makeup that conjure the element of heat and flame. Do you want to look ethereal or otherwordly? Invoke air. Choose clothing, accessories, and makeup that conjure the element of wind, from breeze to storm.
- **Connect with color.** Choose clothing, accessories, and makeup that conjure the power of color and connect with the characteristics you wish to convey. Red for boldness and passion. Pink for nurturing and caring. Orange for creativity. Yellow for optimism and happiness. Green for nature and freshness. Blue for calm and quiet confidence. Purple for power and mystery. Gray for seriousness. Brown for earthiness and endurance. Black for mystery and elegant containment. White for simplicity, cleanliness, and purity.
- **Dress with texture.** Soft clothing is relaxed and forgiving. Crisp fabrics suggest briskness and readiness. Natural fibers connect you with the earth. Synthetic fibers suggests being self-made. Tight

clothing alludes to self-contained power. Loose clothing reflects being free and comfortable.

- **Speak with symbols.** Choose meaningful makeup, jewelry, and symbols to enhance your appearance and convey your glamour.
- **Idealize yourself.** Allow how you look to hint at the mystery and beauty of who you are. You are much more than what you appear.
- **Don't try too hard.** The secret of glamour is its apparent effortlessness. Relax and enjoy the effect.
- **Say an affirmation aloud as you look into the mirror.** Wave your mascara wand if it helps! Believe it.

Your Word is Your Wand: Mindful Beauty Affirmations

Each day I become more radiant.
Each day I become more confident.
Each day I see myself grow.
I can feel my beauty glowing from within.
I seek out the beauty in myself.
I seek out the beauty in the world around me.
My skin and hair glow.
I feel more beautiful with each day that passes.
I take time to care for myself.
I can feel my eyes shining.
I am proud and forgiving of myself.
I look for the good in myself.
I see the beauty in myself.
I am strong and proud of myself.
I am at peace with myself and my body.
I am at peace with . . .
I am the best age I can be today.
I age more gracefully with every day that passes.
I grow in wisdom and strength.
I am capable and strong.

I am full of kindness.
I am full of wisdom.
My skin is smooth and glowing.
I love the curves of my body.
I love my flaws.
Every day my spirit grows with peace.
I am calm and serene.
I am calm and beautiful.
I love how I look.
I look this way to please me.
Each day I see more beauty in the world.
I treat my body with kindness and respect.
I am at peace.
I see beauty.
I feel beautiful.

In Mindful Beauty Treatment 13, did you think of a mindful beauty affirmation that is right for you? Sometimes a personalized affirmation is the magic spell.

Take a Spell: Mindful Beauty Cues
Mindfulness works best in daily activities that are specific and regular. It also helps if they are repetitive, so the more boring the better!

Cue practicing your favorite mindful beauty treatment, such as deep breathing, fully focusing on the task, taking turns to engage one of your five senses, or noticing five things, while you carry out any of the following daily tasks.

- brushing your teeth
- fixing your hair
- applying sunscreen
- massaging in hand lotion

- washing your hands
- checking your makeup
- applying lipstick, gloss, or balm
- spraying on perfume or body spray
- freshening your breath
- filing your nails
- applying moisturizer
- powdering your nose

Make a repetitive self-care task a regular mindful mini break in your daily routine. Use the moment to say a mindful beauty affirmation.

Quick Lift: Impermanent Frown

Becoming more mindful reminds us that everything changes. Nothing stays the same, including our emotions, minds, faces, and bodies. When we embrace the impermanence of our existence, we begin to enjoy it more. We accept uncertainty, movement, and flow. We no longer struggle against a wave in our hair any more than we would struggle against a wave in the ocean. Make a small change in your appearance or self-care routine that makes you look and feel better. Change is beautiful.

The Secrets of Mindful Beauty

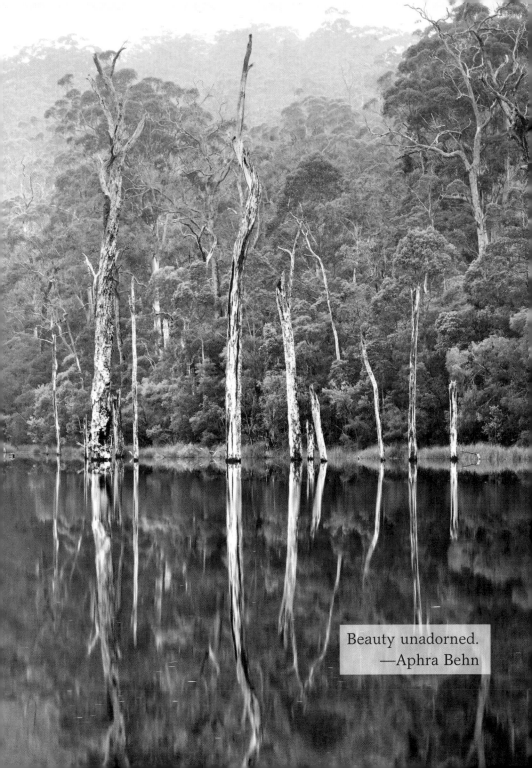

Beauty unadorned.
—Aphra Behn

19 Your Beautiful Nature: Noticing What Is Around You

For centuries, women have connected the natural world with beauty rituals. From ancient times, many beauty practices have taken place outdoors, especially around midsummer, to make the most of the natural light. These old rites invoke many natural elements. They have included collecting particular plants and flowers, using seasonal ingredients in aromatic lotions and health-enhancing potions, washing in clear streams or the morning dew, or arising before dawn to welcome the sun.

Spending time in the natural world is a key element of mindful beauty. You don't need to get up at dawn to bring the beauty of nature into your day. Simply slow down. Take a breath of fresh air before you enter a building. Walk on the sunny side of the street. Stop and look at a flower blooming or a leaf falling. Let raindrops land on your skin, and let the wind blow through your hair. Watch an insect, a bird, or an animal. Go barefoot once in a while. Take your lunch or a meeting to a park instead of an office.

The more often you allow yourself these moments, the more you will seek them out. The more you connect to the beauty of the natural world, the more you will connect to the beauty of your own nature.

Eye Bright: Let In the Light

Bring the natural world into your regular beauty routine. Bring a plant into your beauty space and attend to it every day. Add an element of nature to your dressing table or bathroom counter, such as a polished stone, a fir cone or piece of wood, a seashell or sea glass. Let it be a daily reminder. Before you begin your morning beauty routine each day, take a look out the window. What do your eyes alight upon—snowflakes, raindrops, sunshine? Whatever you see, you are part of it. It's part of you.

Seeing the world in a natural light can change how we perceive it. Natural light boosts our spirits and our well-being. Seasonal affective disorder (known as SAD) is a form of depression that worsens in the wintertime and can be treated by light therapy. Sunshine also boosts our vitamin D levels and our mood. Natural light is also one of the best lights in which to put on makeup. Let there be natural light. Let it stream into your soul.

Psyche: Watching Your Beautiful Mind

The word *psyche*—from which we get *psychology* and *psychiatry*—comes from the Greek, meaning mind or spirit; it also means butterfly.

Your mind is a beautiful butterfly. Watch it for a while, just as you might watch a real butterfly. It might flutter about, land on a flower, soar fast, or glide slow. You might catch it for a moment in the net of your consciousness, or it might elude you.

Be gentle and quiet as you watch your mind, just as you would a real butterfly. Don't disturb it. Observe where it goes without judgment. You don't judge a butterfly for where it lands or how it flies. You don't criticize it. Watch your own mind with the same detachment, appreciation, and interest. See the wonder of it. Don't try to change it. This is a simple method of getting to know your own nature and the nature of your mind.

Watching your own mind is a reminder that you can act as both the observer and the observed. You don't have to be inside your thoughts all the time. If you need relief or just some space from your thoughts, you can step outside and watch them for a moment, even if that moment is as brief as the flutter of a butterfly wing.

This simple exercise is effective at any time. Step back. Close your eyes. Observe the nature of your thoughts. Appreciate the beauty of the butterfly in you.

Open-Minded: Get Fresh

As we become more attuned to the natural world, we notice more. We begin to freshen up, appreciate the newness, growth, and potential around us and in us. Outdoors, we might notice a new bud, a flower opening, or a patch of blue sky. So it is with our own minds. The more attuned we become to our minds, the more easily we remain fresh and open-minded. We might begin to see regular patterns and flight paths we customarily follow. We might notice emotions and body sensations that precede or accompany these thoughts. We might notice that we don't like where our thoughts take us. We might begin to bring more choice into where we take out thoughts, and where they take us.

Choice is a benefit of mindfulness. As we become more self-aware, we make more choices about where we choose to put our attention. It might be challenging at first. Take it easy. Our steps may be tentative on new paths. For a while, we may remain on familiar byways. Then we may become more adventurous and open-minded. We might even be surprised. We can be kind and considerate to ourselves in this process, accepting of the many paths we can choose to take.

Where will your mind take you today?

Beauty Is Every Step: Walking Meditation

This active meditation is practiced outdoors.

Start this meditation by standing still for a moment and tuning in to your breath. Allow yourself to take in a deep, calming breath of outdoor air, feeling the breath travel through your nostrils and down into your lungs. Feel how your stomach expands and contracts. Perhaps you are noticing that the outside air feels crisper or fresher. Perhaps it is warm, heated by the sun. Notice the quality of the air around you. Is there a scent on the air that you didn't notice before? Breathe it in.

Start walking, perhaps a little more slowly than usual. As you walk, allow your attention to shift to your whole body. Feel your legs as they move, the slight swing of your arms. Perhaps you notice how your breath changes slightly as your body starts to move. Notice the sensations of movement, perhaps feeling the wind touching your skin or ruffling your clothes slightly. Feel the ground underneath you, paying attention to the sensation of it traveling through your feet. Is it hard or soft? Is the surface uneven or smooth? Does it change over time as you continue walking?

Tune in to the sounds around you. Can you hear the wind, birds, or cars moving past you? Try to let the sounds find you, noticing them, rather than judging or being affected by them. Notice the sounds you make as you walk, listening to the rhythm of each footstep.

Shift your attention to what you can see. Take in the colors around you, examine the color of the sky, and the colors and tones of the ground. Looking around you, what colors stand out? What shapes? Watch as the prospect before you slowly shifts as you walk, allowing your attention to shift with it.

Now, focus on something in the distance in front of you. As you walk toward it, pay attention to the detail in it. It could be anything— a tree, a signpost, a patch of ground. Notice how at this moment you are experiencing it differently, even if it is something you have walked by many times before. Perhaps you are seeing some beauty in it that you might otherwise have missed. Try this with another object ahead of you, repeating the process as often as you like.

As you end your walk, tune in to your breathing once again. Perhaps your breath is a little faster than it was at the beginning of your walk. Perhaps your chest and stomach feel warmer. Fill your lungs with a final breath of fresh, outdoor air. Imagine that with this breath you are breathing in all the natural beauty you experienced while you walked. As you let the breath out, be mindful of how you can keep these qualities within you wherever you go next.

Quick Lift: Encounter Naked Reality

Do you wear makeup every day? Or do you go bare-faced? Whatever your habit or preference, mix it up. If you wear a lot of makeup try going without for a day. See if it changes your perception of yourself. If you wear little or no makeup, wear more makeup for a day. When you remove it at the end of the day, see if you perceive yourself in a new way. Face your ever-changing reality.

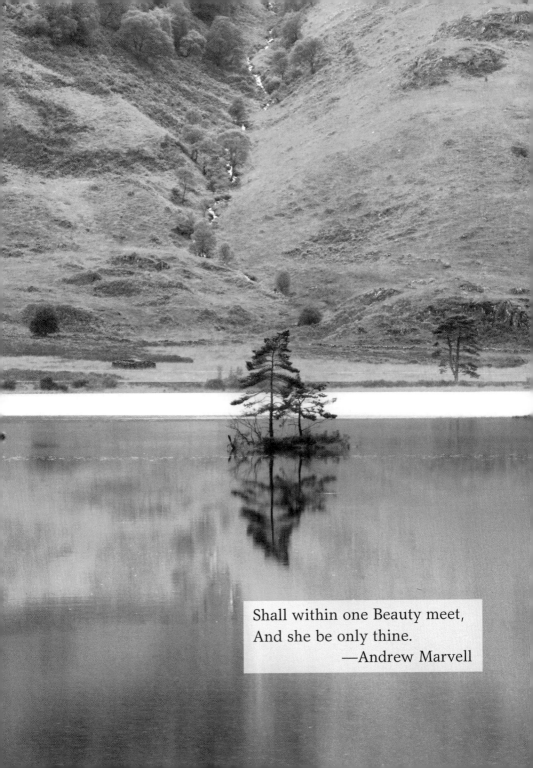

Shall within one Beauty meet,
And she be only thine.
                    —Andrew Marvell

20 Daily Devotions to Beauty

Morning Reflection and Recollection

Recollection is a method used in meditation training and many spiritual traditions. It refers to the gathering up of your thoughts through attention and concentration to transform them into a powerful intention. Recollecting is also a spiritual practice. A *collect* is a form of ancient prayer still used today.

Start your day with a beautiful intention.

Stand in front of a mirror and take a moment to study your reflection. Close your eyes and breathe deeply, concentrating your mind. Open your eyes to your reflection. Read or recite the following meditation:

> *On this day, I resolve to see beauty.*
> *I see beauty within. I see beauty without.*
> *I see beauty in nature. I see beauty in man- and woman-made things.*
> *I see beauty in others. I see beauty in myself.*
> *I create beauty in my mind. I create beauty in my heart.*
> *I create beauty in my body.*
> *Today, I intend to feel beautiful, sense beauty, and think*
> *beautiful thoughts.*
> *This is a beautiful gift I share with others and give myself.*

Coming Home to You Transformation
Welcome home.

One of the descriptions of mindfulness is that it is like coming home to yourself. You will know this from practicing the techniques in this book. A final way to experience this sense of coming home to yourself each day is to engage in a simple mindful beauty homecoming ritual.

The transition between home and work, day and night, is a special time of transformation. When you come home from work or any other activity, take some time to slip into a more comfortable frame of mind.

Depending on how much time you have available, take up one or more of these daily homecoming practices:

- Change your shoes. An old Buddhist tradition is to leave your shoes outside the door of a temple. Take off your work shoes, especially if they are high heels, and put on some footwear that is especially for inside your home. Make it comfortable and beautiful.
- Change your clothes. Take off your workday outer self. Active wear, loose clothing, a robe, or even your pajamas can make you feel relaxed and cherished.
- Turn on a soft light. Whatever the season, switch on a lamp or light a candle rather than just relying on overhead lighting.
- Cleanse your hands. Do this mindfully. Think about washing away the debris of the day.
- Remove or touch up your makeup. Some evenings you may like to remove it; sometimes you might simply want to freshen up.
- Smile and say "welcome home" to yourself in the mirror. Reconnect to your breath home base.

Home Base Meditation
Sit in a comfortable, quiet place. Take up your meditation posture, keeping your spine straight. Don't slouch or curl your body.

Gently close your eyes and begin to focus on your breathing. Direct your attention to your breath home base. This is your nose, mouth, throat, chest, diaphragm, or belly. Feel the breath going in and out of that part of your body. Notice the sensation. Explore it. Rest your attention in that part of your body. Mentally put your feet up after a long day. Breathe in and out a few times. If your attention wanders, gently return home when you are ready to do so.

As you breathe, say the word *home* as you exhale. It sounds a bit like "ommm." This sound is comforting to many people. Repeat the word *home*—to yourself or out loud—as many times as you choose.

Stay at home base for as long as you wish.

Gently open your eyes.

Visiting your breath home base is a lovely meditation to do regularly. You'll find the way home faster the more you practice. It only takes a few minutes to sit in your favorite meditation posture and really come home to you. You'll soon notice that you feel much more centered, calm, and happy at home.

Your breath home base is portable. Once you know where your breath home base is located in your body, you'll be able to find it more easily wherever you are. You can access it in other places too, at work, when traveling, or while socializing. Take yourself to a quiet place and go home. Sit, stand, or lie down, whatever is accessible to you. After you've made a trip to your breath home base, you'll return refreshed.

Mindfulness meditation helps us to direct our attention where we want it to go. The more you rest your attention in your breath home base, the easier you will find it comes back during meditation and whenever you want to direct your attention in your life (away from unwanted thoughts or emotions) or better concentrate. Your home base is waiting to welcome you. Come and go as you please.

Like Dorothy in *The Wizard of Oz*, there's no place like home. Make your way to your home base, your breath center, wherever you are, at whatever time of day. When we connect to our breath home base, we don't even need to tap our heels together. We can always go home.

Evening Reflection and Recollection

Gratitude is a beautiful emotion. Giving daily thanks for all the beauty and good in the world is a transformative practice.

The aim of old collects was to gather up the prayers of the people. Collects remind us that our desires—health, safety, peace, prosperity, love, and beauty—are both singular and universal. We are one of a kind, yet one of many. Recollecting brings us into a fuller experience of the world and our place in it.

End your day with gratitude.

Standing in front of a mirror, take a moment to study your reflection. Close your eyes and breathe deeply, concentrating your mind. Open your eyes to your reflection. Read or recite the following meditation:

I give thanks for this beautiful day.
I give thanks for the beauty I have encountered and shared.
For beauties seen by my eyes, thought by my brain, and felt
in my heart,
For all beauty seen and unseen, known and unknown, I give thanks.
May my awareness expand to appreciate more forms of beauty
in the world.
May all beings be cherished and recognized as beautiful.
May this night bring peaceful slumbers and beautiful dreams to all.

Commit to Self-Care

Self-care takes commitment. It's all too easy to start a new routine, diet, or exercise program and then let your good intentions fall by the wayside.

Make a mindful commitment to self-care. Insert your own name and repeat the following:

"I, _____, mindfully commit to caring for myself. For richer or poorer, in sickness and in health, from this day forward, I will love, honor, and cherish my physical and psychological beauty and well-being."

Quick Lift: Practice Makes No Need to Be Perfect

Mindful beauty isn't about perfection. It's about accepting ourselves, how we look, how we feel, and the world around us, as it is right now. That's good news if your inner perfectionist is aiming to do mindfulness perfectly. You can't! It's not possible! The more you practice mindfulness, the better you will get at it – that's guaranteed. But you'll never be perfect at mindfulness. You'll only become more accepting and comfortable with imperfection. That's so much better than trying to be perfect. Keep practicing, and may you always enjoy the process.

The Secrets of Mindful Beauty

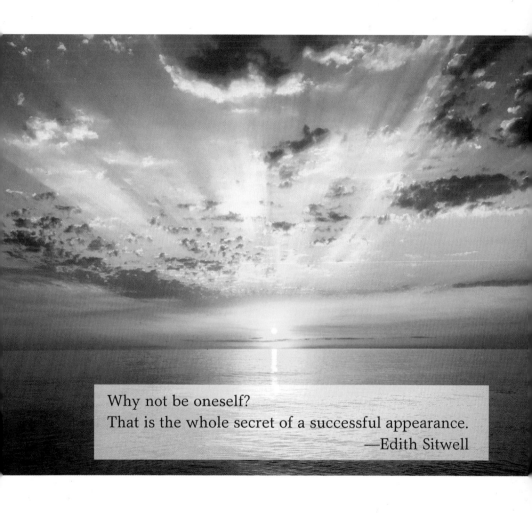

Why not be oneself?
That is the whole secret of a successful appearance.
—Edith Sitwell

The Mindful Beauty Treatments

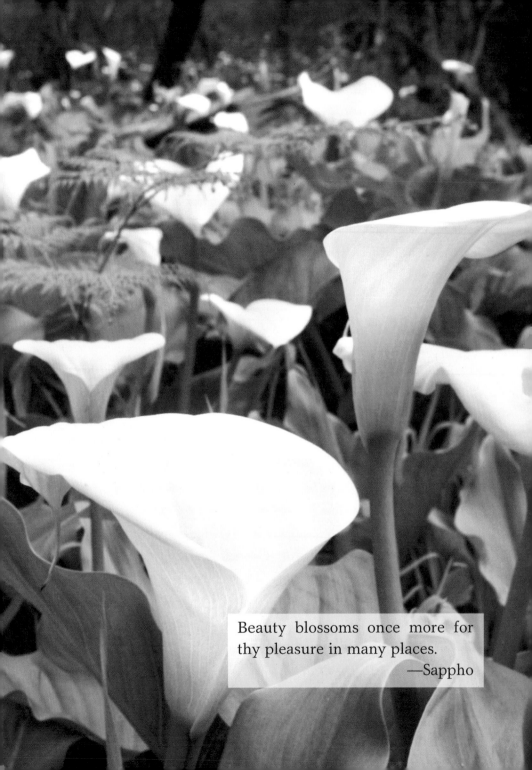

Beauty blossoms once more for thy pleasure in many places.

—Sappho

Conclusion

Go with Grace: The Virtue of Beauty

Beauty is a virtue. That's what the ancient Greeks and Romans believed. Beauty was considered both a spiritual and physical expression, a form of grace. Being full of grace was viewed as a quality of expression, of character, not merely a bodily attribute. We recognize grace. It is radiant; we are drawn toward it. Grace lights up our faces; it lights up the world.

Grace is greater than appearances. It adds up to more than the sum of its parts. It's an expression of the whole person, body and soul. The most beautiful face in the world can be spoiled by an unkind expression. Beholding real beauty goes deeper. It turns and guides us toward what is worth seeking in our lives. Our behaviors and expressions all lend themselves to beauty, if we mind them.

Practicing mindfulness is a way of cultivating grace. Self-care can be considered a form of daily ethics, of practicing the virtue of beauty. Sharing beauty, in all its diversity, with ourselves and others is a moral responsibility. We never have to apologize for it. Beauty is an attitude, a philosophy. When we behave beautifully, we bring grace into our minds, our faces, and into the world.

At different times in our lives, we may choose different methods to enhance and improve our appearance. But without the gifts of grace—self-awareness, acceptance, kindness, compassion—we'll only scratch the surface. Mindful beauty takes us deeper. Loving who we are, as we are right now, at this moment in time, will give us clear skin, a bright smile, and sparkling eyes for life. Aging gracefully is truly mind over matter.

Let your beauty shine through no matter what age you are. May your mind, body, and spirit be full of grace.

Stay mindful. Stay beautiful.

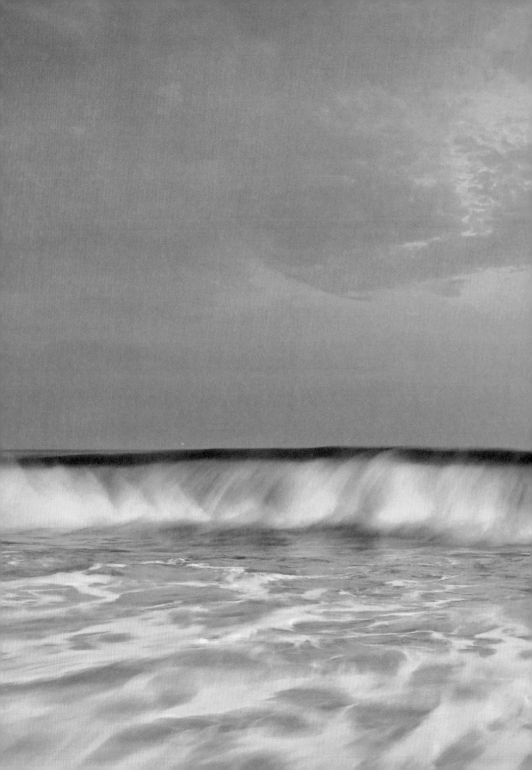

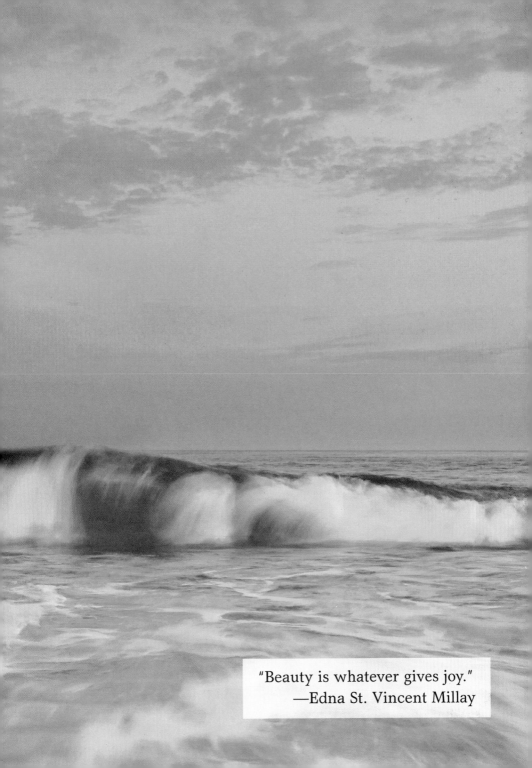

"Beauty is whatever gives joy."
—Edna St. Vincent Millay

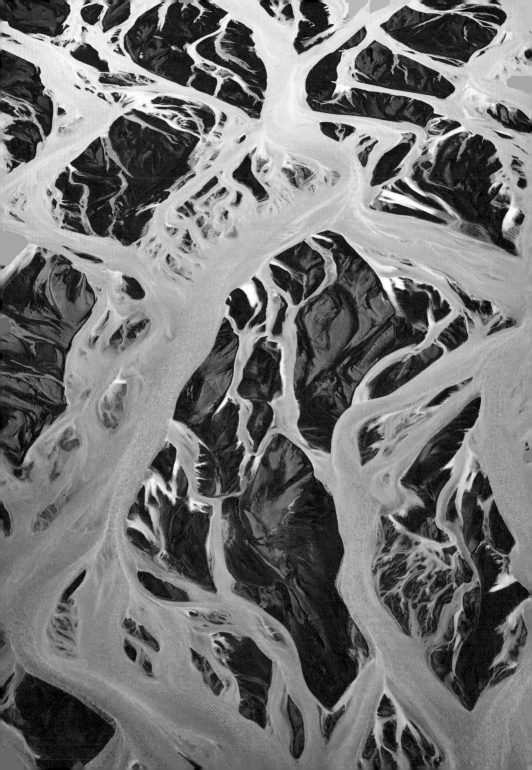

Bibliotherapy

Books (and other resources) to improve your mindfulness!

Family Favorites

- *Mindfulness for Beginners* (2006) by Jon Kabat-Zinn (Sounds True, 2006) is one of the recent classics of mindfulness literature. It offers a collection of reflections and practices that can be explored at random or as a daily primer. Kabat-Zinn is one of the leaders of mindfulness in psychology and the founder of mindfulness-based stress reduction (MBSR), which emphasizes the value of coming back to our bodies and our senses over and over again. His book *Wherever You Go, There You Are* is another great read.
- *Counterclockwise: A Proven Way to Think Yourself Younger and Healthier* by Ellen Langer (Hachette, 2009). Ellen Langer is called the mother of mindfulness. *Counterclockwise* explores mindfulness, health, and aging and greatly influences our approach. Her classic *Mindfulness* (now in a twenty-five-year anniversary edition) is a guide how to avoid living a "mindless" life governed by unthinking habits and routines, and her book *On Becoming an Artist* connects mindfulness and creativity.

- *The Miracle of Mindfulness: The Classic Guide to Meditation by the World's Most Revered Master* by Thich Nhat Hanh (Ebury Publishing, 2008) is a premier Buddhist guide to the practice. It explains how simple acts like washing the dishes or drinking tea can be transformed into acts of meditation. Thich Nhat Hanh's poetry is also a useful meditative starting point. His *Peace is Every Step* inspired our idea of beauty in every step.
- *The Happiness Trap* by Russ Harris (Exisle, 2013) is written by a leader in acceptance commitment therapy (ACT), a mindfulness-based program to help us accept all of who we are and how we feel—the good, the bad, the ugly, and the beautiful. One of Jessica's top recommendations.
- *Mindfulness: A Practical Guide for Finding Peace in a Frantic World* by Mark Williams and Danny Penman (Hachette, 2011) focuses on mindfulness-based cognitive therapy (MBCT) and provides useful mindfulness meditations. Audio, video, and a workbook are also available. MBCT is particularly helpful for depression.
- *Flourish: A Visionary New Understanding of Happiness and Well-being* by Martin E. P. Seligman (Free Press, 2011). We are big fans of Martin Seligman, the founder of the positive psychology movement, from his work on learned helplessness versus learned optimism to how we can thrive and not just survive in life.
- *The Power of Now* by Eckhart Tolle (Namaste, 2004) is an example of popularizing the concept of mindfulness into an accessible format and language. We particularly recommend his practical approach in the associated workbook.
- Shinzen Young is the meditation master Elizabeth first followed to learn Buddhist meditation. Simple, soothing, and effective, his excellent range of audio meditation guides, including *The Beginner's Guide to Meditation*, are available via Sounds True.
- UCLA Mindfulness meditation podcasts. These excellent podcasts are a terrific guide and introduction to the technique from the

UCLA Mindful Awareness Research Center. Other resources are available too. We use these podcasts regularly.

- *Whispers of Spirit, Whispers of Healing,* and *Whispers of Now* are among a series of whispered meditations for those who find silent meditation too deafening or challenging. People with anxiety may especially appreciate this method. Available from Sounds True with original soundtracks by Brian Scott Bennett.

- Pema Chodren is a Tibetan Buddhist nun, teacher, and author. Her many books and audio guides to Buddhist practice are engaging and accessible. Elizabeth particularly likes *Getting Unstuck: Breaking Your Habitual Patterns and Embracing Naked Reality* (audio, Sounds True, 2005).

- *Practical Mysticism* by Evelyn Underhill (first published 1915). An old guide to meditation and contemplation from the Christian perspective that complements and enhances mindfulness.

- *A Guide for the Advanced Soul* by Susan Hayward (DeVorss & Co., 2010). We have a few copies of these calligraphic quotations and affirmations in our family. We think it might have inspired Jessica to give her father a box of her own handwritten affirmations as a birthday gift when she was about ten years old.

- *Starbright: Meditations for Children* by Maureen Garth (HarperCollins, 1991). Simple, soothing meditations and visualizations to help sleep, awaken creativity, and increase concentration. These beautiful meditations were how Jessica was introduced to meditation as a child.

- *Seeking Sophia* by Josephine Griffiths (Millenium Books, 1997). A spiritual guide with reflections and meditations for women. Elizabeth has been fortunate enough to have the author's personal direction for many years, and we have both attended her silent retreats. A gem.

- *Look Younger, Live Longer* by Gayelord Hauser (Faber and Faber, 1950). This vintage book took Hollywood by storm and inspired the Cranks whole food restaurants in the UK. Elizabeth's grandmother shared its philosophy. This Gayelord, nutritionist and self-help author, was before his time (and the Focker movies!).

- *The Art of Extreme Self-Care* by Cheryl Richardson (Hay House, 2013). Elizabeth is on her third copy of this book, having given the previous two away to family members! She also recommends it to her university students.

Selected Resources and References

APMNA (Association for Psychoneurocutaneous Medicine of North America). (n.d.). Retrieved December 16, 2015, from http://www.psychodermatology.us/

Axmar, E. (2016). *Mindfulness: The Mindfulness Meditation Guide for a Mindful and Stress-Free Life.* Author.

Baer, R. A. (Ed.). (2015). *Mindfulness-Based Treatment Approaches: Clinician's Guide to Evidence Base and Applications.* London: Academic Press.

Bewley, A., Taylor, R. E., Reichenberg, J. S., and Magid, M. (Eds.). (2014). *Practical Psychodermatology.* Oxford: Wiley.

Bishop, S. R., Lau, M., Shapiro, S., Carlson, L., Anderson, N. D., et al. (2004). Mindfulness: A proposed operational definition. *Clinical Psychology: Science and Practice, 11*(3), 230–241.

Block-Lerner, J., Adair, C., Plumb, J. C., Rhatigan, D. L., and Orsillo, S. M. (2007). The case for mindfulness-based approaches in the cultivation of empathy: Does nonjudgmental, present-moment awareness increase capacity for perspective-taking and empathic concern? *Journal of Marital and Family Therapy, 33*(4), 501–516.

Bochun, P. (2011). Mindfulness and creativity. *Canadian Teacher Magazine,* (Nov/Dec), 8–9.

Brown, B. (2010). *The Gifts of Imperfection: Let Go of Who You Think You're Supposed to Be and Embrace Who You Are.* Center City, MN: Hazelden.

Carmody, J., and Baer, R. A. (2008). Relationships between mindfulness practice and levels of mindfulness, medical and psychological symptoms and well-being in a mindfulness-based stress reduction program. *Journal of Behavioral Medicine, 31*(1), 23–33.

Carney, D., Cuddy, A. and Yap, A. J. (2010). Power posing: Brief nonverbal displays affect neuroendocrine levels and risk tolerance. *Psychological Science (21)*10, 1363–1368. doi:10.1177/0956797610383437

Casey, John. (1990). *Pagan virtue: An essay in ethics.* Oxford: Clarendon Press.

Claxton, G. (2005). Mindfulness, learning and the brain. *Journal of Rational-Emotive and Cognitive-Behavior Therapy, 23*(4), 301–314.

Clay, R. A. (2015). The link between skin and psychology. *Monitor on Psychology 46*(2), 56. Retrieved December 16, 2015, from http://www.apa.org/monitor/2015/02/cover-skin.aspx

Crane, R. (2008). *Mindfulness-Based Cognitive Therapy.* London: Routledge.

Day, A. M. (2013). *Mindful Living: Workbook and Journal for Life Transformation.* Bloomington, IL: Author House.

Deyo, M., Wilson, K. A., Ong, J., and Koopman, C. (2009). Mindfulness and rumination: Does mindfulness training lead to reductions in the ruminative thinking associated with depression?. *EXPLORE: The Journal of Science and Healing, 5*(5), 265–271.

Eskenazi, L. (2007). *More Than Skin Deep: Exploring the Real Reasons Why Women Go Under the Knife.* New York: Harper Collins.

Etcoff, N., Orbach, S., Scott, J., and D'Agostino, H. (2004). The real truth about beauty: A global report. Findings of the global study on women, beauty and well-being. Retrieved February 23, 2010, from: http://www.campaignforrealbeauty.com/uploadedFiles/dove_white_paper_ final. pdf

Germer, C. (2004). What is mindfulness. *Insight Journal, 22,* 24–29. Retrieved from http://www.drtheresalavoie.com/userfiles/253125/file/insight_germermindfulness.pdf

Goldfaden, G., and Goldfaden, R. (2010). Getting your beauty sleep with topical melatonin. *Life Extension Magazine.* Retrieved from http://www.lifeextension.com/magazine/2010/4/Getting-Your-Beauty-Sleep-with-Topical-Melatonin/Page-01?p=1

Hagen, A. (2007). *The Yoga Face: Eliminate Wrinkles with the Ultimate Natural Facelift.* New York: Penguin.

Hanh T. N. (1975). *The Miracle of Mindfulness: An Introduction to the Practice of Meditation.* Boston: Beacon Press.

Hanh, T. N. (1988). *The Sun My Heart: From Mindfulness to Insight Contemplation. London: Rider.*

Hanson, R. (2011). *Just One Thing: Developing a Buddha Brain One Simple Practice at a Time.* Oakland: New Harbinger Publications.

Jafferany, M. (2011). Psychodermatology: When the mind and skin interact. *Psychiatric Times, 28*(12), 1–2. Retrieved from http://pro.psychcentral.com/psychodermatology-when-the-mind-and-skin-interact/00710.html

Kabat-Zinn, J. (2011). *Mindfulness for Beginners: Reclaiming the Present Moment—and Your Life.* Boulder: Sounds True.

Kabat-Zinn, J. (2013). *Full Catastrophe Living: Using the Wisdom of Your Body and Mind to Face Stress, Pain, and Illness.* New York: Random House.

Kabat-Zinn, J., Massion, A. O., Kristeller, J., Peterson, L. G., Fletcher, K. E., et al. (1992). Effectiveness of a meditation-based stress reduction program in the treatment of anxiety disorders. *American Journal of Psychiatry, 149*(7), 936–943.

Kang, C., and Whittingham, K. (2010). Mindfulness: A dialogue between Buddhism and clinical psychology. *Mindfulness, 1*(3), 161–173.

Kersting, K. (2003). Psychodermatology's first postdoc. *Monitor on Psychology 34*(8), 34. Retrieved December 16, 2015, from http://www.apa.org/monitor/sep03/postdoc.aspx

Kuyken, W., Watkins, E., Holden, E., White, K., Taylor, R. S., et al. (2010). How does mindfulness-based cognitive therapy work? *Behaviour Research and Therapy, 48*(11), 1105–1112.

Lau, M. A., Segal, Z. V., Witkiewitz, K. A., and Marlatt, G. A. (2007). Mindfulness-based cognitive therapy as a relapse prevention approach to depression. In K. A. Witkiewitz and G. A. Marlatt (Eds.), *Therapist's Guide to Evidence-Based Relapse Prevention* (pp. 73–90). Burlington, MA: Academic Press.

Le Minhluan. *Drink your tea - Tea meditation (poem by Thich Nhat Hanh)* [video]. Retrieved from https://www.youtube.com/watch?v=ZVPZZOLi3w4

Lowen, A. (2004). *Narcissism: Denial of the True Self.* New York: Simon and Schuster.

Ma, S. H., and Teasdale, J. D. (2004). Mindfulness-based cognitive therapy for depression: Replication and exploration of differential relapse prevention effects. *Journal of Consulting and Clinical Psychology, 72*(1), 31–40.

Neff, K. D., Kirkpatrick, K. L., and Rude, S. S. (2007). Self-compassion and adaptive psychological functioning. *Journal of Research in Personality, 41*(1), 139–154.

Oprah Winfrey Network. *Thich Nhat Hanh's Tea Meditation | Super Soul Sunday | Oprah Winfrey Network* [video]. Retrieved from https://www.youtube.com/watch?v=LNiwOI0u9AI

Piet, J., and Hougaard, E. (2011). The effect of mindfulness-based cognitive therapy for prevention of relapse in major depressive disorder: A systematic review and meta-analysis. *Clinical Psychology Review, 31*(6), 1032–1040.

Reb, J., Narayanan, J., and Chaturvedi, S. (2014). Leading mindfully: Two studies on the influence of supervisor trait mindfulness on employee well-being and performance. *Mindfulness, 5*(1), 36–45.

Richards, M. (1997). *Opening Our Moral Eye.* Hudson, NY: Lindisfarne Books.

Rose, P. (2002). The happy and unhappy faces of narcissism. *Personality and Individual Differences, 33*(3), 379–391.

Salovey, P., Rothman, A. J., Detweiler, J. B., and Steward, W. T. (2000). Emotional states and physical health. *American Psychologist, 55*(1), 110–121.

Sanford, L. T., and Donovan, M. E. (1984). *Women and Self-Esteem: Understanding and Improving the Way We Think and Feel About Ourselves.* London: Penguin Books.

Schonert-Reichl, K. A., and Lawlor, M. S. (2010). The effects of a mindfulness-based education program on pre- and early adolescents' well-being and social and emotional competence. *Mindfulness, 1*(3), 137–151.

Shapiro, J. (2007). Hair loss in women. *New England Journal of Medicine, 357*(16), 1620–1630.

Stahl, B., and Goldstein, E. (2010). *A Mindfulness-Based Stress Reduction Workbook.* Oakland: New Harbinger Publications.

Teasdale, J. D., Segal, Z. V., Mark, J., Ridgeway, V. A., Soulsby, J. M., et al. (2000). Prevention of relapse/recurrence in major depression by mindfulness-based cognitive therapy. *Journal of Consulting and Clinical Psychology, 68*(4), 615–623.

Turner, J. (2015). *The Fringe Hours: Making Time for You.* Grand Rapids, MI: Revell.

Twenge, J. M., and Campbell, W. K. (2009). *The Narcissism Epidemic: Living in the Age of Entitlement.* New York: Atria Paperback.

Williams, J. M. (2008). Mindfulness, depression and modes of mind. *Cognitive Therapy Research*, *32*(6), 721–733.

Williams, M., and Penman, D. (2011). *Mindfulness: An Eight-Week Plan for Finding Peace in a Frantic World*. New York: Rodale.

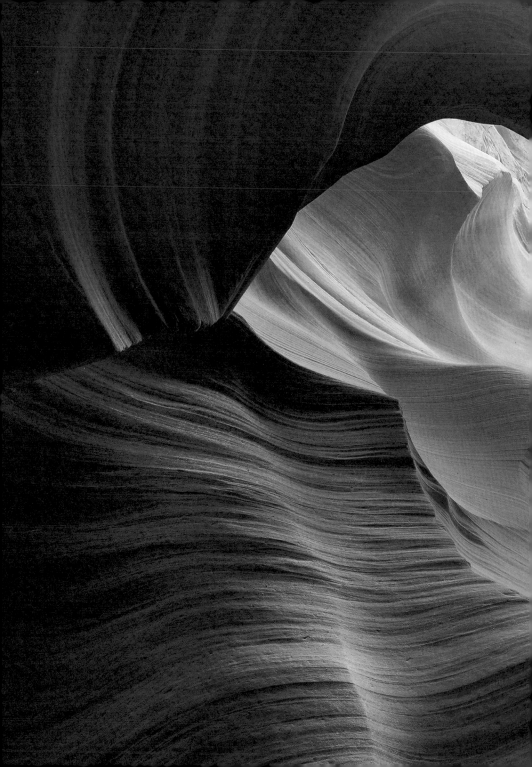

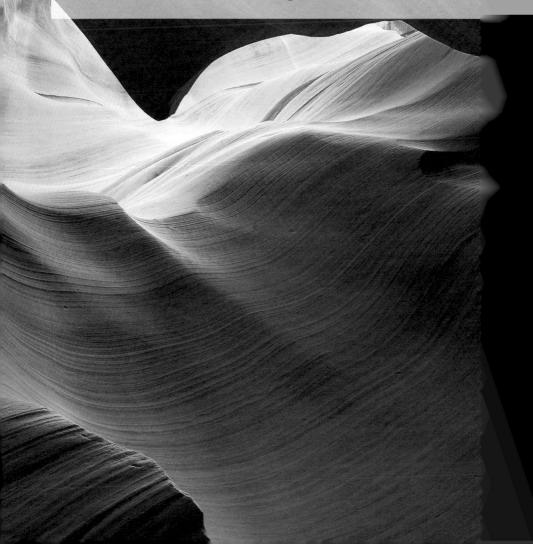

Don't keep *Mindful Beauty* a secret!
Visit Elizabeth and Jessica at www.mindfulbeauty.net
or find them on Facebook, Instagram, or Twitter.
Join a community of beautifully minded people!

The beautiful photographs in this book were taken by
international photographer Steve Fraser. To see more,
visit his website at http://stevefraser.co

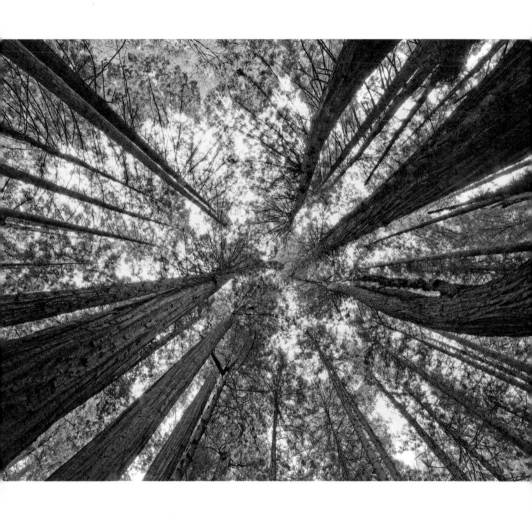

Acknowledgments

The authors would like to thank the inspirational Steve Fraser for the opportunity to work with him; their wonderful agent, Joelle Delbourgo, for her support and encouragement; and everyone at Skyhorse Publishing, especially Brooke Rockwell, who made this book so beautiful.

About the Authors

Elizabeth Reid Boyd (Bachelor of Science, Doctor of Philosophy) age 48

Dr. Elizabeth Reid Boyd has degrees in psychology and gender studies. She has taught interpersonal communication and personal development skills for almost two decades. She is an academic at Edith Cowan University and has lectured in Australia and Singapore. She is coauthor of *Body Talk: A Power Guide for Girls*. Elizabeth also writes fiction under the name Eliza Redgold, based upon the Gaelic meaning of her name. She has published romances internationally with Harlequin, and her historical fiction *NAKED: A Novel of Lady Godiva* was published by St. Martin's Press.

Jessica Moncrieff-Boyd (Bachelor of Arts, Master of Clinical Psychology, Doctor of Philosophy) age 28

Jessica Moncrieff-Boyd is an emerging researcher and practitioner in the field of psychology. She completed her undergraduate degree at the University of Melbourne, majoring in psychology and creative writing, and undertook a combined Masters/PhD in clinical psychology at the University of Western Australia. Jessica is a recipient of an Australian postgraduate award and has been a visiting researcher at the University of Exeter, UK. She has published in the areas of eating disorders and body image.

Inspired by *Mindful Beauty*, the mother-daughter pair practice what they preach and love to share it.